Vit Mi and Dietary Supplements

Written for
The American Dietetic Association
by Marsha Hudnall, MS, RD

CHRONIMED PUBLISHING

Vitamins, Minerals, and Dietary Supplements: Up-to-Date Tips
on Getting the Essential Nutrients You Need From the World's
Foremost Experts on Nutrition. © 1999 by The American Dietetic
Association.

Originally published as *Vitamins, Minerals, and Food Supplements*
© 1996 by The American Dietetic Association.

Library of Congress Cataloging-in-Publication Data

Vitamins, minerals, and dietary supplements / The American
Dietetic Association

    p.   cm.

Includes index.

ISBN 1-56561-170-5

Edited by: Jeff Braun
Cover Design: Terry Dugan Design
Text Design & Production: David Enyeart
Art/Production Manager: Claire Lewis

Printed in the United States of America

Published by
Chronimed Publishing
P.O. Box 59032
Minneapolis, MN 55459-0032

.**NOTICE: CONSULT A HEALTH CARE PROFESSIONAL** Readers are advised to
seek the guidance of a licensed physician or health care professional
before making changes in health care regimens, since each individual
case or need may vary. This book is intended for informational purposes
only and is not for use as an alternative to appropriate medical care.
While every effort has been made to ensure that the information is
the most current available, new research findings, being released with
increasing frequency, may invalidate some data.

Vitamins, Minerals, and Dietary Supplements

Written for The American Dietetic Association by
Marsha Hudnall, MS, RD
Nutrition, Health, &
   Fitness Communications
Ludlow, Vermont

The American Dietetic Association Reviewers:
Diane W. Heller, MMsC, RD
Nutrition Plus
Marietta, Georgia

Cheryl L. Rock, PhD, RD, FADA
The University of Michigan
Ann Arbor, Michigan

Jean Schoen, RD
National Center for Nutrition
   and Dietetics
Chicago, Illinois

Technical Editor:
Betsy Hornick, MS, RD
The American Dietetic Association
Chicago, Illinois

CHRONIMED PUBLISHING

THE AMERICAN DIETETIC ASSOCIATION is the largest group of food and health professionals in the world. As the advocate of the profession, the ADA serves the public by promoting optimal nutrition, health, and well-being.

For expert answers to your nutrition questions, call the ADA/National Center for Nutrition and Dietetics Hot Line at (900) 225-5267. To listen to recorded messages or obtain a referral to a registered dietitian (RD) in your area, call (800) 366-1655. Visit the ADA's Website at www.eatright.org.

Contents

Introduction

NUTRITION HAS GRABBED THE ATTENTION of health-conscious individuals like no other time before. People everywhere are trying to extend and improve the quality of their lives by turning to good nutrition. Not only does it fuel today's activities, it helps set the stage for a healthy, active future.

Headlines, however, often make it seem like there is controversy about how to reach those goals. But the truth is, there is no question about the first and foremost nutritional strategy: To promote health and reduce your risk of chronic disease eat a balanced diet that includes a wide variety of foods. Do this and most people can obtain the essential nutrients—in the proper amounts—and help secure a foundation for good health.

Still, many people look to dietary supplements, hoping for an extra advantage in the quest for good health. A dietary supplement is any product taken by mouth that contains "dietary ingredients." These ingredients may include vitamins, minerals, herbs or botanicals, enzymes, amino acids, or other substances used to supplement the diet. They come in various forms, such as pills, tablets, capsules, liquids, or powders. What supplement makers claim their products do, also runs the gamut.

For example, one dietary supplement is touted as nature's most perfect food, able to boost energy and cure impotence. Another supplement treats baldness, lowers blood cholesterol, and controls weight, says its manufacturer.

Be aware that many of the claims for dietary supplements

are unproven. This fact, however, holds little sway with some people. In fact, when steps were taken to better regulate these claims, the Food and Drug Administration (FDA) was bombarded with millions of letters and faxes in protest! In part, people were reacting to unfounded fears that medical prescriptions would be needed to obtain vitamin, mineral, and other supplements. And even though the regulations are intended only to help better inform and protect the public, many consumers have demanded an almost "hands-off" policy regarding dietary supplements.

Later in this book, we'll discuss the regulations. For now, though, the experience simply shows the intense interest in vitamin, mineral, and dietary supplements. Indeed, surveys show four out of ten Americans regularly used dietary supplements in the early to mid-1980s. And a 1993 *Newsweek* poll found seven out of ten of people use supplements at least occasionally. Approximately 3,400 different vitamin and mineral supplements are currently sold, generating $4 billion in sales annually. In 1994, the government even established an Office of Dietary Supplements at the National Institutes of Health to coordinate research on dietary supplements and disease prevention.

Is all this interest warranted? Do you truly need vitamin, mineral, and dietary supplements for good health? The answer depends on three factors: your usual food choices, whether you face particularly high nutrient needs for any reason, and whether you are following a diet for medical or other purposes that limits nutrient intake.

In general, a balanced and varied diet supplies all the vitamins and minerals you need. But there are circumstances where supplements are both effective and safe. This book reviews those circumstances as well as other important information necessary to decide whether you need vitamin, mineral, or other dietary supplements. It also provides information to help you choose a supplement, should you or your health care provider decide you need one. Also of note: Specific information for each vitamin and mineral, including recommended or safe amounts, appears in the Appendices.

As you will learn, vitamins and other supplements can be a piece of the healthful equation for many people, but they are not the only answer.

So, while this book is titled *Vitamins, Minerals, and Dietary Supplements,* we hope it also spurs you to consider your entire diet and all the parts of your life that impact your health.

Chapter One
Eating for Good Health

AS WE ENTER THE 21ST CENTURY, more and more attention is being paid to the role of vitamins and minerals in preventing chronic diseases. This isn't too surprising when you consider that nutritionists in the early 1900s were also looking for ways to prevent disease; however, their focus was different. They spent much of their time helping people get enough nutrients, including vitamins, to prevent deficiency diseases. Although our bodies need only very small amounts of vitamins, people at that time frequently lacked vital nutrients. They suffered diseases such as beriberi (a deficiency of thiamin), scurvy (a deficiency of vitamin C), and pellagra (a deficiency of niacin).

With today's abundant food supply, it's much easier to eat a varied diet and obtain the recommended amounts of vitamins and minerals. Because of this, nutrition issues related to the effects of too much food or certain nutrients have taken the forefront in recent years. For example, scientists are investigating the impact of eating too many calories on our risk for certain types of cancer. Likewise, too much saturated fat in the diet has been linked to heart disease—the #1 killer in this country. In the case of dietary supplements, we know that too much of one vitamin or mineral may affect the absorption and utilization of another, creating imbalances that may harm your health.

Even so, there's evidence that we continue to fall short in other nutrition areas, and it goes beyond just missing out on specific food components. Research suggests our failure to eat enough of whole groups of food ranks as one of the most significant contributors to our risk for chronic diseases. We'll explain.

Foods such as grains, whole grains, fruits, and vegetables contain a host of nutritious substances, including carbohydrates, protein, vitamins, minerals, fiber, and phytochemicals (biologically active compounds in plant foods linked to good health). While each of these substances plays a specific role in good health, together they provide the best defense against disease.

For example, an adequate intake of vitamin C helps the white blood cells fight off infections. Protein, however, plays an equally vital role. It enables the body to make antibodies. Separately, vitamin C and protein help keep us healthy. But it takes both nutrients (along with others found in a healthful diet) to foster an optimally-functioning immune system that can ward off illnesses. That's why a healthful diet or eating style should be your starting point for guarding your health through nutrition.

How Our Diets Measure Up

You don't have to just take our word for it when we say food provides the nutrients in the amounts most of us need every day. National surveys prove it.

The National Health and Examination Survey is a periodic assessment of our diets conducted by the federal government. It compares people's diets to the Recommended Dietary Allowances (RDAs). The RDAs were first published in 1943 as a guide for the amounts of specific nutrients healthy individuals need to consume to prevent deficiency problems. Since then, the RDAs have been revised periodically to reflect our growing knowledge regarding the need for different nutrients. More recently, new intake guidelines called Dietary Reference Intakes (DRIs) have been released to update RDAs for certain nutrients. You may now see recommendations referred to as RDA levels or as Adequate Intake (AI) levels. No matter which term is used—RDA or AI—it represents the best available estimate of intake for optimal health.

The closer your diet comes to supplying nutrients in amounts listed in the RDAs, the greater the likelihood you are meeting your nutrient needs. Conversely, the further your intake falls below the RDAs, the greater the chances that you are not getting the nutrients you need for good health. (See Appendices 1 and 2 for the complete listing of RDAs and AIs, along with specific, summarized information about each nutrient.)

The third and most recent National Health and Examination Survey is encouraging. It shows on average that we're easily meeting the RDAs for most vitamins and minerals with what we get from food. In only a few cases—such as calcium, folate, and iron intakes in women—does our typical intake fall short of recommended amounts. Even so, by following the advice to eat foods rich in those nutrients, you can easily get enough.

The following table shows you how the diets of a 40 to 49 year old woman and a 30 to 39 year old man compare with recommendations for several vitamins and minerals.

	40–49 Year-Old Woman		30–39 Year-Old Man	
	RDA	**Avg. Intake**	**RDA**	**Avg. Intake**
Vitamin A	800 RE*	829 RE*	1000 RE*	1245 RE*
Vitamin C	60 mg	88 mg	60 mg	123 mg
Thiamin	1.1 mg	1.33 mg	1.2 mg	2.06 mg
Riboflavin	1.1 mg	1.59 mg	1.3 mg	2.47 mg
Niacin	14 mg	19.25 mg	16 mg	29.71 mg
Calcium	1000 mg	685 mg	1000 mg	1049 mg
Iron	18 mg	12.05 mg	10 mg	19.16 mg
Folate	400 mcg†	180 mcg	400 mcg	359 mcg
Vitamin B$_{12}$	2.4 mcg	3.79 mcg	2.4 mcg	7.34 mcg

*retinol equivalents
†micrograms

Source: *Dietary Intake of Vitamins, Minerals, and Fiber of Persons Ages 2 Months and Over in the United States: Third National Health and Nutrition Examination Survey, Phase 1, 1988–91*, Advance Data, Number 258, November 14, 1994, National Center for Health Statistics, Hyattsville, MD.

The Basics of Healthy Eating

The Dietary Guidelines for Americans feature seven strategies you can use to eat healthfully (see below). By following these guidelines, healthy adults and children (2 years and older) can enjoy better health and reduce their chances of developing serious problems such as heart disease and certain types of cancer. Developed jointly by two government agencies—the U.S. Departments of Agriculture (USDA) and Health and Human Services (DHHS)—the guidelines represent the most up-to-date advice from nutrition scientists about healthful eating.

The Dietary Guidelines focus on the total diet—that is, the nutritional quality of all the foods you eat put together—rather than individual foods. This allows for a wide variety of eating styles and choices that bring pleasure as well as health to eating.

While the Dietary Guidelines recognize the importance of vitamins and minerals to meet special nutritional needs, they emphasize that supplements cannot take the place of proper food choices. Plain and simple, a pill or other type of supplement cannot supply all of the vitamins, minerals, and other substances in foods that are important to health. Further, when higher amounts of vitamins and minerals are recommended, many experts say we should get them from fortified foods. These foods provide the benefits of extra nutrients along with healthful substances found naturally in the food.

The Dietary Guidelines for Americans

➤ Eat a variety of foods.
➤ Balance the food you eat with physical activity—maintain or improve your weight.
➤ Choose a diet with plenty of grain products, vegetables, and fruits.
➤ Choose a diet low in fat, saturated fat, and cholesterol.
➤ Choose a diet moderate in sugar.
➤ Choose a diet moderate in salt and sodium.
➤ If you drink alcoholic beverages, do so in moderation.

Source: *Nutrition and Your Health: Dietary Guidelines for Americans*, Fourth Edition, 1995, USDA and USDHHS.

To help you better select foods and design an overall eating plan to meet the Dietary Guidelines, the USDA and DHHS also developed the Food Guide Pyramid (below). The Pyramid is an outline of what to eat each day, not a rigid prescription. It calls for eating a variety of foods to get the nutrients you need while supplying the right amount of calories to help you maintain a healthy weight.

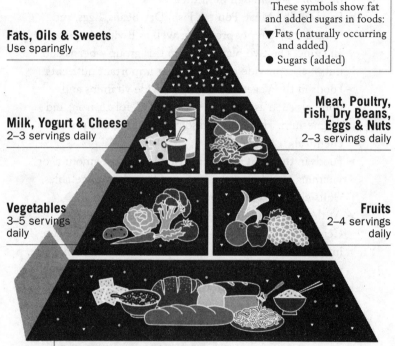

These symbols show fat and added sugars in foods:
▼ Fats (naturally occurring and added)
● Sugars (added)

Fats, Oils & Sweets
Use sparingly

Meat, Poultry, Fish, Dry Beans, Eggs & Nuts
2–3 servings daily

Milk, Yogurt & Cheese
2–3 servings daily

Vegetables
3–5 servings daily

Fruits
2–4 servings daily

Breads, Cereals, Rice & Pasta
6–11 servings daily

The Pieces of the Pyramid

The Food Guide Pyramid emphasizes foods from five major food groups. Each of these groups provides some, but not all, of the nutrients you need. That means foods in one group can't replace those in another. What's more, no one food group is more important than another; for good health, you need them all.

➤ The tip of the Pyramid shows fats, oils, and sweets. These include foods such as salad dressings and oils,

Eating for Good Health

cream, butter, margarine, sugars, soft drinks, and candies. These foods provide calories but few vitamins, minerals, or other nutritionally beneficial substances. Most people should use them sparingly.

➤ Foods in the Milk, Yogurt, and Cheese Group are important sources of protein, vitamins, and minerals. In particular, they're rich in calcium, a mineral many people don't get enough of in their diets.

➤ Foods in the Meat, Poultry, Fish, Dry Beans, Eggs, and Nuts Group supply protein as well as B vitamins, iron, and zinc. The two plant foods in this group—beans and nuts—also provide fiber and other important nutrients.

➤ Foods in the Vegetable Group provide vitamins and minerals such as vitamin A, vitamin C, folate, iron, and magnesium. These foods also contain fiber and phytochemicals.

➤ Foods in the Fruit Group provide important amounts of vitamins A and C, potassium, and fiber. Like vegetables, fruits also contain phytochemicals.

➤ At the base of the Food Guide Pyramid are Breads, Cereals, Rice, and Pasta—all foods from grains. They are important sources of complex carbohydrates, vitamins, minerals, and phytochemicals. You need the most servings of these foods each day. Choose at least three servings of whole grains daily for the extra vitamins, minerals, fiber, and phytochemicals they contain.

The Food Guide Pyramid also features a range of servings from each food group. How many servings you need each day depends on your calorie needs. Almost everyone should have at least the lowest number of servings in the ranges. See "How Many Calories are Right for You?" and "How Many Servings Do You Need?" (page 17) for more information.

To keep fat intake within recommended limits, choose low-fat foods from each group most of the time. Also moderate your use of added fats such those found in the Pyramid tip.

How Many Servings Do You Need?

	Daily Calorie Needs		
	About 1600	About 2200	About 2800
Bread Group Servings	6	9	11
Vegetable Group Servings	3	4	5
Fruit Group Servings	2	3	4
Milk Group Servings*	2–3	2–3	2–3
Meat Group (ounces)	5	6	7

. . . .

How Many Calories are Right for You?

Your calorie needs depend on your age, sex, size, and how active you are.

➤ 1600 calories is about right for many sedentary women and some older adults.

➤ 2200 calories meets the needs of most children, teenage girls, active women, and many sedentary men. Women who are pregnant or breastfeeding may need more. Preschool children need the same variety of foods as older family members, but may need less than 1600 calories. For fewer calories, they can eat smaller servings, although they need the equivalent of 2 cups of milk each day.

➤ 2800 calories is about right for teenage boys, many active men, and some very active women.

Women who are pregnant or breast-feeding, teenagers, and young adults to age 24 need 3–4 servings.

Adapted from *The Food Guide Pyramid*, Human Nutrition Information Service, U.S Department of Agriculture, Home and Garden Bulletin Number 252, August 1992.

. . . .

Chapter Two

Vitamins and Minerals

Mighty Micronutrients

WHILE THE IMPORTANCE OF FOOD to health has long been recognized, it has only been in the last 100 years that we've known about vitamins—even that they existed! Since then, we have discovered the essential role vitamins play in preventing deficiency diseases such as scurvy, rickets, some types of anemia, even night blindness.

We've been aware of the importance of many minerals in the diet for much longer. But in just the past 25 years, our understanding of how both vitamins and minerals work has increased dramatically (although we still have a lot to learn!). For example, we now know they may also play a part in preventing the diseases that currently take the most toll on Americans' health, such as heart disease, cancer, and osteoporosis.

Even so, we're still working to understand how specific vitamins and minerals work individually and together to protect health. The following gives a brief overview of vitamin and mineral basics, and Appendices 1 and 2 explain in more detail the vitamins and minerals we know the most about.

Vitamins 101

Vitamins and minerals are also called micronutrients because we need them in only tiny amounts. But those small amounts play powerful roles! They work with other nutrients to help your body perform the many functions that keep you going each day.

For example, many vitamins help regulate bodily processes,

partnering with substances to facilitate necessary chemical reactions in your body. Minerals work similarly in many cases. They also serve more familiar roles such as forming the basic substance of teeth and bones.

Vitamins are divided into two groups: water-soluble and fat-soluble. The group name describes how they are carried in food and transported in the body.

Water-soluble vitamins include vitamin C and the B-vitamins: thiamin (B_1), riboflavin (B_2), niacin, vitamin B_6, folate, vitamin B_{12}, biotin, and pantothenic acid. Fat-soluble vitamins include vitamins A, D, E, and K.

Focus on...Antioxidants If nutrition headlines grab your eye when perusing the newspaper, you've no doubt already read plenty about the potential benefits of antioxidant vitamins and minerals. Claims for these "wonder" nutrients abound, from preventing heart disease and cancer to even slowing down the natural processes of aging!

Is there any basis for these claims? If so, how much do you need to take full advantage of their benefits? First, let's look at how antioxidants work.

While oxygen is necessary to life, it also has its down side. When oxygen is burned in the cells, oxygen byproducts called free radicals are produced. Free radicals can damage body cells, as well as DNA. DNA contains the body's master plan for reproducing cells—damage may change the "directions" it gives, resulting in abnormal, unhealthy cells. Other factors, such as cigarette smoke, burns, and ultraviolet light, also cause free radicals to form in the body.

The damage caused by free radicals can lead to problems such as cancer, heart disease, cataracts, and the deterioration that goes along with aging. But antioxidants can neutralize free radicals before they have a chance to cause harm. They may even help undo some of the damage already done to body cells.

Antioxidant nutrients include three micronutrients: beta carotene (other carotenoids may be protective, too), vitamin C, and vitamin E. Several minerals also contribute to antioxidant activities in the body: selenium, copper, zinc, and manganese. While they each perform separate functions—vitamin C, for example, removes free radicals from cell fluids, and beta carotene and vitamin E work within body fat—they seem to complement each other. That means we need them all for best results.

How do you get them all? A balanced diet based on the Food Guide Pyramid is your best bet for several reasons. First, research has linked diets rich in fruits and vegetables with lower rates of health problems such as heart disease, high blood pressure, and cancer. But it's not yet clear which components of these foods provide disease-preventing benefits. It may be the antioxidants they contain, other phytochemicals, or something else altogether.

It is clear, however, that antioxidant supplements will not replace diets rich in fruits and vegetables. Studies have shown that taking large amounts of beta carotene supplements may not provide any benefits, and could even cause harm. Likewise, in one study of heavy smokers, vitamin E supplements did not influence the risk of developing cancer or dying from any specific cause, but were linked to more cases of a certain type of stroke.

The bottom line: Supplements cannot substitute for a diet rich in fruits and vegetables. Although antioxidants alone may not prevent diseases, foods rich in antioxidants clearly offer protective health benefits. Beta carotene-rich foods include sweet potatoes, carrots, pumpkin, apricots, peaches, cantaloupes, and spinach.

Foods rich in vitamin C include oranges, grapefruits, peppers, cantaloupe, strawberries, potatoes, kale, and other foods. For vitamin E, choose plant foods such as nuts, seeds, and vegetable oils. Fortified cereals and green leafy vegetables such as mustard and turnip greens, kale, and collards are good low-fat sources of vitamin E. See Appendix 2 on pages 93–104 for more foods rich in antioxidant minerals.

Mineral Basics

Minerals are another group of important nutrients. They are necessary to help body chemical reactions and processes take place as well as to provide structure (in the form of bones and teeth, for instance). Minerals make up only about 4 percent of your weight, but they are a part of every body tissue. Undoubtedly, they're essential to life!

The "major" minerals include those we need the most of—calcium, phosphorus, magnesium, sodium, chloride, and potassium. The last three are called electrolytes; together they help regulate fluid in the body and transmit nerve, or electrical, impulses.

Other minerals we need in much smaller amounts—less than 20 milligrams a day compared to the 250 or more milligrams we need of the major ones. These "trace" minerals include chromium, copper, fluoride, iodine, iron, manganese, molybdenum, selenium, and zinc.

Only a few of the trace minerals have RDAs set at this point: iron, zinc, iodine, fluoride, and selenium. Until we learn more, a range of "Estimated Safe and Adequate Daily Dietary Intakes" are given for the rest.

Several other trace elements have been identified, including tin, arsenic, silicon, vanadium, nickel, and boron. But at this point, little is known about their role in human health, or how much the body needs, if any. As a result, neither RDAs nor "safe and adequate" ranges are specified for these elements.

Like vitamins, minerals are transported and stored in your body in different ways. Some minerals travel through the bloodstream to reach the areas they're needed, and any excess passes out in urine or feces. Others attach to body proteins and become part of the body structure. As a result, excessive amounts may be harmful. See Appendix 2 on page 93 to learn more about these essential nutrients.

Focus on...Calcium We've got more calcium in our bodies than any other mineral—and about 99 percent of it is in our bones. If we don't get enough calcium, that's where it shows!

We need plenty of calcium for strong, healthy bones. Because calcium is necessary for several body processes, if you don't get enough of it, your body draws calcium from your bones. If that happens too often—or if you don't get enough calcium when your bones are growing or don't absorb or use the calcium you do get (due perhaps to deficiencies of other nutrients such as vitamin D)—it can set you up for osteoporosis later in life. Osteoporosis is one of the leading causes of disability in this country. It is characterized by weak and fragile bones and is responsible for back pain and hip fractures as well as "Dowager's hump." Inadequate calcium may also be linked to other problems, such as colon cancer, high blood pressure, and preeclampsia (high blood pressure during pregnancy).

The best time for building bones is during childhood and teen years, but peak bone mass continues to build until age 35. After then, bones begin to slowly lose calcium as a natural part of the aging process. Women experience the largest losses during and after menopause, when estrogen levels drop. Estrogen protects bones during child-bearing years.

To protect against osteoporosis and other problems associated with an inadequate calcium intake, follow these tips:

➤ Consume enough calcium. Revised recommendations for calcium intake were recently released. For several age groups, the recommended amounts have increased. See Appendix 2, page 94, for specific requirements for each age group.

➤ The preferred source of calcium is calcium-rich foods such as dairy products. The Food Guide Pyramid recommends 2 to 3 servings per day of dairy foods, and 3 to 5 servings per day of vegetables. One cup (eight ounces) of milk contains approximately 300 milligrams of calcium. Green vegetables such as broccoli, kale, turnip greens, and Chinese cabbage contain less, but can contribute significantly to total calcium intake. Some vegetables such as spinach, rhubarb, chard, and beet greens contain oxalic acid, which binds with calcium in the digestive tract to produce calcium oxalate. This form of calcium is not well-absorbed.

➤ If you are lactose intolerant (cannot digest milk sugar), you may be better able to tolerate yogurt with live, active enzymes, aged cheese, or milk treated with lactase (an enzyme). You may also be able to tolerate milk in small amounts and with other foods.

➤ People who limit their intake of dairy foods, such as certain vegetarians, can obtain calcium through green vegetables (see above); tofu processed with calcium; some legumes; fish canned with bones; seeds; nuts; and fortified foods such as fortified soy milk, juices, drinks, breads, and cereals. See "Vegetarian Diets," page 40.

➤ Calcium supplements are preferred by some people. Absorption is best when taken in single doses of 500 milligrams or less and when taken with meals.

➤ Calcium citrate, another type of calcium supplement, may be better absorbed than calcium carbonate by older people who have reduced amounts of stomach acids.

➤ If you also take iron supplements, take them at different times of the day than calcium supplements. They're each better absorbed when taken on their own.

➤ Avoid calcium supplements that contain dolomite, oyster shell, or bone meal. They may also contain lead and other undesirable metals.

➤ Purchase supplements that will dissolve in the stomach (see "Getting What You Pay For," page 60).

➤ Consume enough vitamin D. Vitamin D is required to absorb calcium. See Appendix 1 on page 81 for food sources of vitamin D.

➤ Get enough exercise—at least three times weekly. Regular, weight-bearing activities, such as walking, strength-training, dancing, and tennis, stimulate bone formation.

➤ Avoid smoking and excessive amounts of alcohol.

Focus on...Iron It's ironic. Although iron is widely distributed in foods, and you need only small amounts to stay healthy, iron deficiencies are common everywhere in the world, even the United States. And that's no small problem. A shortfall of this important mineral can lead to anemia and its symptoms: fatigue, weakness, and poor health. Iron also helps to keep your immune system operating at peak efficiency.

Why is iron so important? Its major job in the body is to carry oxygen to the cells to make energy. So it makes sense that if you don't have enough iron, you may feel tired and just not at your best.

The need for iron is highest during periods of rapid growth, child-bearing years for women, and pregnancy (see "The Child-

Turn to the Label

Where can you go for quick and easy information on the vitamin and mineral content of foods? The "Nutrition Facts" panel—required on all packages of prepared foods. It lists the content per serving of at least four vitamins and minerals: vitamin A, vitamin C, calcium, and iron. Manufacturers can also include other vitamins and minerals in the food, which they'll likely do if the food is a good source. Amounts are listed as "% Daily Values," a figure that tells you how much one serving of the food contributes to the daily total recommended intake of a nutrient (see page 27). For tips on reading the "Supplement Facts" panel, see page 57.

Bearing Years," page 36). Women who have undergone menopause, and men need less iron than other groups of people.

In most people, the body has a built-in mechanism for getting the iron it needs while avoiding excesses: When iron stores are low, absorption rises. When iron stores are adequate, absorption slows.

Another important factor is the type of iron eaten: heme iron or non-heme iron. While both types are important sources of the mineral, heme iron found in foods of animal origin such as meats is better absorbed than non-heme iron from plant sources. But you can enhance your ability to absorb non-heme iron by consuming it with foods high in vitamin C or with foods that contain heme iron.

One final point about iron: The question whether too much iron may be linked to problems such as heart disease and cancer has recently received a lot of attention. Free iron in the body can potentially damage cells, much like free radicals can (see "Focus on...Antioxidants," page 20). But the body normally keeps most of its iron stored away where it can do no harm. More research is needed before we can definitely say there's a link.

There is a real risk, however, for people who inherit a gene that causes the body to absorb too much iron. As many as one out of every 250 Americans is at risk for this problem, called hemochromatosis. Men and postmenopausal women, whose iron needs are low, run the highest risk of developing symptoms of this serious disease. The disease, in which iron builds up in the body and causes tissue damage, can lead to arthritis, diabetes, and heart irregularities. Symptoms include fatigue, bronze skin discoloration, abdominal pain, and achy joints.

The best way to test for hemochromatosis is through blood tests. The only way to get rid of excess iron if you have hemochromatosis is through regular blood donations.

Eating a balanced diet based on the Food Guide Pyramid is the best nutrition advice for people at risk for hemochromatosis. Such a diet moderates meat, fish, and poultry, which contain well-absorbed heme iron. Iron supplements are definitely not recommended.

What's in a Name? If you've tried to stay nutrition savvy over the years, you might be a bit confused about the standards used to measure the vitamin and mineral content of foods and dietary supplement products. With various terms for nutrient standards, like RDAs (Recommended Dietary Allowances), DVs (Daily Values), and now DRIs (Dietary Reference Intakes), you might even suspect a conspiracy to confuse! Rest assured, it just represents an ongoing effort to provide consumers with useful information to judge the nutrient content of a food or a supplement.

At this point, when reading nutrition labels on foods and supplements, you can forget all terms except Daily Values. These reference values were established for use in nutrition labeling. The DVs for vitamins and minerals are based on the RDAs, and are average allowances for nutrients (often the highest RDA amount) that meet the varying needs of all persons aged four and older. These allowances may exceed minimum requirements of nutrients for some people, but are established to be adequate to meet the needs of practically all healthy persons. The "% DV" for a vitamin or mineral listed on a nutrition label tells you how much one serving of that food or supplement contributes towards the average daily requirement for that vitamin or mineral.

The following gives the actual amount of vitamins or minerals that 100 percent of the DV provides. If you've been advised to take more of a particular vitamin or mineral, you would need more than 100 percent of the DV. For example, if you need 1300 milligrams (1.3 grams) of calcium daily, you would need 130 percent of the DV. Nutrients from a variety of foods, and supplements if needed, can add up to supply what you need.

What Does 100% of the Daily Value Equal?

Vitamin/Mineral	Daily Value
Vitamin A	5000 IU
Vitamin C	60 mg
Vitamin D	400 IU
Vitamin E	30 IU
Vitamin K	80 mcg
Thiamin	1.5 mg
Riboflavin	1.7 mg
Niacin	20 mg
Vitamin B_6	2 mg
Folate	400 mcg
Vitamin B_{12}	6 mcg
Biotin	0.3 mg
Pantothenic acid	10 mg
Calcium	1000 mg
Iron	18 mg
Phosphorus	1000 mg
Iodine	150 mcg
Magnesium	400 mg
Zinc	15 mg
Copper	2 mg
Selenium	70 mcg
Manganese	2 mg
Chromium	120 mcg
Molybdenum	75 mcg
Chloride	3400 mg

Source: U.S. Food and Drug Administration

Words Count

Food and supplement manufacturers may tout the nutritional benefits of their products, but how they do it is scrutinized. For instance, if a claim such as "High in folate" is made on the label, folate must also be featured on the Nutrition Facts or Supplement Facts panel. The same is true when other vitamins or minerals are specifically mentioned on a product label. And claims that foods or supplements are "good sources," "rich in," or otherwise special sources of an approved nutrient, such as vitamins and minerals, must meet strict government regulations. For more on reading supplement labels, see Chapter 4.

What Label Claims Mean*

More, Fortified, Enriched, Added Contains at least 10 percent more of the Daily Value, compared to the reference food

Good Source, Contains, Provides 10 to 19 percent of the Daily Value

High, Rich In, Excellent Source of 20 percent or more of the Daily Value

---

*Per standard serving size (Reference Amount). Some claims have higher nutrient levels for main dish products and meal products, such as frozen dinners and entrées. For more information, call or write the food manufacturer.

....

Kitchen Savvy—Preserving Nutrients in Foods

The way you store and prepare food can destroy vitamins before they ever make it into your body. Although hardier, minerals can be lost, too. Follow these simple tips for preserving the vitamins and minerals in your food.

➤ Store fresh and canned fruits and vegetables in cool places. Some vitamins are sensitive to heat. Cook vegetables for the shortest time possible, to a crisp, tender stage, in a covered pot.

➤ Steam or microwave vegetables in as little water as possible. Both vitamins and minerals can seep into cooking water. If you have to use a lot of water, such as when boiling potatoes, save it to make soup or sauce later.

➤ If vegetables must be cooked for a long time, cut them in

the largest pieces possible to expose fewer surfaces to water and heat.

> Keep the skins intact on fruits and vegetables. Peeling not only removes the nutrients concentrated just under the skin but also exposes oxygen-sensitive nutrients such as vitamin C.

> Do not add baking soda to protect the green color of vegetables; this destroys vitamins. Instead, cook only as long as necessary.

> Do not use copper or brass cooking utensils, which can destroy vitamin C.

> Store milk in opaque or cardboard containers to protect from light, which destroys riboflavin.

In this chapter, we've covered the importance of vitamins and minerals, how they work individually and together to protect health. As you know, for most healthy people, a balanced diet based on the Food Guide Pyramid is the best source for nutrients. At the same time, there are circumstances where a vitamin and/or mineral supplement may be needed. In the next chapter, we will examine if supplements are right for you.

Chapter Three
Should You Take One?

THERE'S NO QUESTION that a pill cannot substitute for a healthy diet. But are there any instances in which a healthy diet may not supply all the vitamins and minerals you need?

The best way to answer that question is to examine the various circumstances or situations that people face during their lifetimes that may call for extra vitamins or minerals, or for which claims have been made that extra vitamins or minerals are needed.

In general, it comes down to this: Multivitamin/mineral supplements that provide no more than 100 percent of the Daily Value (DV) may be beneficial for people who:

➤ have limited dietary intakes, or

➤ have special needs due to other factors, or

➤ just don't eat a well-balanced diet.

Multivitamin/mineral supplements may not provide an advantage to people who eat according to the Dietary Guidelines. What's more, it is possible that even small amounts of extra vitamins or minerals may contribute to excessive intakes or imbalances. Still, the rule in deciding whether to take a supplement is to examine your situation to determine whether you may benefit.

Determining Your Need for Vitamin or Mineral Supplements

Take this quick quiz to determine whether you should consider supplements. Check the statements that apply to you. A check does not automatically mean you need a supplement. Read the section in this book that discusses the impact of your circumstance or habit on your vitamin and mineral needs. If you need more help, or if you have a concern that's not discussed in this book, contact a registered dietitian. He or she can help you decide the best nutritional strategy for you.

___ 1. I tend to skip meals. See page 40.

___ 2. I eat fewer than 5 servings of fruits/vegetables and 3 servings of whole-grain foods every day. See page 15.

___ 3. I don't get a lot of variety in my diet. For example, I only eat one or two kinds of vegetables most of the time. See page 11.

___ 4. I completely avoid whole groups of foods, such as meat, poultry, and fish or milk and milk products. See page 40.

___ 5. I avoid all foods of animal origin. See page 40.

___ 6. I'm a teenager. See page 34.

___ 7. I'm of childbearing age, or am already pregnant or breast-feeding. See page 36.

___ 8. I take oral contraceptives. See page 39.

___ 9. I'm female, past menopause, and not on hormone replacement therapy. See page 39.

___ 10. I'm over 50. See page 34.

___ 11. I take a variety of medicines (either prescription or non-prescription). See page 49.

___ 12. I don't drink milk, nor do I get out in the sun much. When I am out, I use lots of sunscreen. See page 22 and Appendix 1, page 79.

___ 13. I have a poor appetite. See page 40.

___ 14. I just don't have time to eat balanced meals. See page 40.

___ 15. I'm constantly dieting to control my weight. See page 39.

___ 16. I'm scheduled for, or recovering from, surgery or other physical injury. See page 47.

The Age Factor

Vitamin and mineral supplements may be needed at some times in your life more than others—simply because of your age. Read on for guidelines.

Infancy. All newborns should receive an injection or oral dose of vitamin K immediately following birth. After that, whether you should supplement your baby's diet with vitamins and minerals depends on if you breast-feed or use formula. No matter what, supplements should never be self-prescribed, but given only with a doctor's or registered dietitian's advice.

Most breast-fed babies should receive vitamin D supplements if exposure to sunlight is limited, as is the case with many infants. After 6 months of age, fluoride supplements should also be given if the fluoride content of your water supply is low. Adequate fluoride helps in the development of cavity-resistant teeth.

After 4 to 6 months of age, breast-fed infants should also get another source of iron, such as iron supplements or iron-fortified cereal. Infants nursed by vegetarian mothers may also need vitamin B_{12} supplements.

If your baby is not breast-fed, he or she should receive iron-fortified formula. Fluoride supplementation may also be necessary after 6 months of age if your local water supply is not fluoridated.

Childhood. Many pediatricians regularly prescribe multivitamin/mineral supplements that contain 100 percent of the DVs for children. But in general, a balanced diet can supply needed vitamins and minerals.

Often the rationale for giving supplements is to provide a sense of assurance that children are getting the vitamins and minerals they need for proper growth. As a parent, though, it may be helpful to realize that a young child's eating habits are typically erratic. Eating "jags" are common, where your child eats only one type of food for several days. It is also not unusual for children to refuse to eat different types of foods. These habits will not likely lead to nutritional deficiencies, but if you are uncertain or have questions, speak with your pediatrician or registered dietitian.

Fluoride supplementation may be advised throughout your child's first eight years to provide the greatest protective effect on dental health. Ask your doctor whether your child should take fluoride supplements. If your water supply is fluoridated, fluoride supplements are not necessary.

Adolescence. By the time many children reach adolescence, independence and changing lifestyles add up to one thing—poor eating habits. It's no wonder: Regular snacking on low-nutrient foods combined with the frequent skipping of well-balanced meals can lead to nutrition gaps. Nutrients that teens often come short on are iron and calcium, especially teen girls. In fact, daily calcium requirements for teens have recently increased to 1300 milligrams—the highest level for any age group.

If you or your teenager is concerned about his or her dietary habits, a multivitamin/mineral supplement that contains no more than 100 percent of the DVs may provide some help—but it won't substitute for healthful eating. And there's more than vitamins and minerals at stake here. Such eating habits also usually mean a diet that is high in fat and low in fiber and other nutrients, which may set the stage for health problems in later years. The best bet is to work towards improving eating habits. If you need help, consult with a registered dietitian.

Over 50. The golden years can present a few situations that may call for vitamin/mineral supplements. If you're taking medications that interfere with the absorption or utilization of vitamins or minerals, a supplement may indeed be necessary. See "Do Medicines Affect Your Vitamin and Mineral Needs?" on page 49, or check with your doctor or pharmacist about your medications.

Calcium is an important mineral for both men and women. After age 50, when the rate of bone loss increases, the recommended intake jumps to 1200 milligrams daily. For women not on hormone replacement therapy—their calcium needs may be even higher because the hormone estrogen is no longer available to help protect bones. If you're an older adult, you may require a calcium supplement to meet your increased needs, especially if milk and dairy products are not a regular part of your diet. (For more on calcium, see "Focus on....Calcium," page 22.)

Likewise, vitamin D supplements may be necessary if you don't consume adequate amounts of vitamin D-fortified foods, such as milk, or you spend most of your time indoors. Because of potential toxicity problems, however, vitamin D supplements should only be taken with the advice of a physician.

As you age, your ability to absorb the naturally occurring form of vitamin B_{12} may become impaired. Therefore, older adults should get most of their vitamin B_{12} from foods fortified with this vitamin, such as most breakfast cereals, or from supplements.

The senses of taste and smell may also decline as we age. That can affect appetite and interest in food, leading to a poor diet. In addition, wearing dentures sometimes causes similar problems, either by interfering with these senses, or because they do not fit well. Problems with depression or eating alone can also lead to reduced food intakes.

In general, however, research has not proven that healthy older people eating balanced diets benefit from vitamin/mineral supplementation. Your decision to supplement should be based on an assessment of your diet by a qualified health professional such as a doctor or registered dietitian. Never self-diagnose a health problem or prescribe your own special diet or dietary supplement.

While supplements won't solve problems that may lead to dietary insufficiencies, a daily multivitamin/mineral that does not exceed 100 percent of the DVs can provide needed nutrients while you work at a real solution.

For Women Only

Several times during their lives, women face an increased need for certain vitamins and minerals. Again, while a balanced diet can generally meet those needs, multivitamin/mineral supplements may be beneficial in special instances.

The Child-Bearing Years. Neural tube defects (NTDs), which include anencephaly and spina bifida, account for about 5 percent of all U.S. birth defects each year. Infants born with anencephaly are missing most or all of their brain and die shortly after birth. Most babies born with spina bifida, in which the spinal cord is exposed, grow to adulthood but suffer severe paralysis or other disabilities.

According to the Centers for Disease Control and Prevention, the incidence of these painfully crippling defects could be cut in half in this country if all women of childbearing age consumed adequate amounts of folate, a B vitamin. In reality, many women do not know exactly when they get pregnant—and the neural tube of a fetus starts forming immediately. Recently released recommendations for folate advise that any woman capable of becoming pregnant (14–50 years) should get 400 micrograms of folic acid daily from foods fortified with folic acid, from vitamin supplements, or a combination of the two. This is in addition to the folate found naturally in certain foods. Folic acid is the "man-made" form of folate found in fortified foods and dietary supplements.

Beginning in January 1998, enriched grain products, including most breads, flour, pastas, rice, and cereals, are required by law to be fortified with folic acid. On the labels of these fortified products, you'll see folate (or folic acid) listed on the Nutrition Facts panel along with its % Daily Value (% DV). The % DV tells you how a serving of the food contributes to your daily needs. To meet the daily requirement of 400 micrograms, the % DV for folate (or folic acid) from your food choices and vitamin supplements over the course of a day should add up to at least 100 percent. Keep in mind that the only foods that contain folate in the form of folic acid are fortified grain products.

Since it is so important to get enough folate even before you know you're pregnant, it may pay to take a multivitamin and mineral supplement—especially if you're planning to become pregnant and you suspect that you're not getting enough from foods fortified with folic acid.

The RDA for iron is also higher during child-bearing years. Still, the need for supplementation with iron depends on your individual needs and eating patterns. For instance, women who experience heavy menstrual bleeding may need to supplement with iron. But the decision to do so should be based on blood tests performed by a physician.

Likewise, due to misconceptions about how to manage their weight or reduce their risk for chronic disease, many women today limit or even entirely avoid particularly good sources of iron such as meats and poultry (especially dark meat). Even so, an iron supplement may not be necessary. Iron can be obtained in adequate amounts from fish and plant sources such as leafy greens, legumes, and enriched or fortified breads and cereals.

To enhance absorption of iron from plant sources, consume a vitamin C-rich food or meat, poultry, or fish with a plant source of iron. To enhance absorption of iron supplements, take them between meals. Some people experience less abdominal discomfort with iron supplements that are time-released.

Pregnancy and Nursing. Once you know you're pregnant, the folate requirement for pregnancy increases to 600 micrograms per day. It's important that at least 400 micrograms come from fortified foods or supplements. The remaining 200 micrograms can come from foods with naturally occurring folate. Most prenatal vitamins meet the requirements for folic acid, but you'll also want to include more folate from your food choices. See Appendix 1 for food sources of folate.

Many obstetricians routinely prescribe prenatal vitamin/mineral supplements to ensure that vitamin and mineral needs are met. However, a report issued by the Subcommittee on Nutritional Status and Weight Gain During Pregnancy of the National Academy of Sciences, advised that evidence does not support routine supplementation with vitamins and minerals other than iron. Still, the report does point out that there clearly are situations in which supplementation may be wise. For example, being a vegetarian or excluding dairy products increases the likelihood that you're not getting enough of certain vitamins and minerals, such as vitamins B_6, B_{12}, D, and folate as well as calcium, zinc, and iron. (See "Vegetarian Diets," page 40.) If the diet cannot be improved, a prenatal supplement may be desirable— but only with the physician's approval. The best advice is to follow your doctor's guidance both in whether you should take any supplements, and if so, how much you should take.

Indeed, physician approval is an absolute must for any supplements taken during pregnancy. A case in point: Studies show that excessive vitamin A poses significant risk for birth defects, especially when taken in the first trimester. Supplements containing preformed vitamin A should only be taken under medical supervision during pregnancy.

Women expecting twins or multiple births may also have higher vitamin/mineral needs that justify supplementation. And pregnant adolescents face a combination of higher vitamin and mineral needs and potentially poor eating habits, warranting a close look at the need for supplementation.

Nursing moms face higher vitamin and mineral needs than usual, but a balanced diet in amounts recommended can easily meet those needs. Still, your dietary choices can mightily affect the bottom line. Trying to lose weight by restricting calories to less than about 1800 calories per day can drive vitamin and mineral intakes down. Milk production may fall as well. Certainly, while a multivitamin/mineral supplement may help, the best strategy is to improve your food choices.

Likewise, avoiding milk and other calcium-rich dairy products may point to the need for a calcium supplement for nursing women. And limited exposure to sunlight and avoidance of vitamin D-fortified milk increases the risk for vitamin D deficiencies. A physician-approved supplement may be necessary.

Vegetarian nursing mothers have special needs, too. See "Vegetarian Diets," page 40.

Premenstrual Syndrome. Supplements of vitamin B_6, vitamin E, and magnesium are sometimes recommended to relieve the symptoms of premenstrual syndrome, which include food cravings, irritability, depression, headache, bloating, and weight gain. But studies have consistently failed to prove these supplements work. Indeed, when vitamin B_6 was given in doses as high as 100 times the RDA, it did not relieve symptoms any more effectively than a placebo. Conversely, there's real risk involved: Large doses of vitamin B_6 can cause nervous system problems. Likewise, too much magnesium can produce a range of undesirable effects.

A higher need for any micronutrients premenstrually has not been identified.

Use of Oral Contraceptives. Using oral contraceptives may increase your need for some vitamins and minerals such as vitamin B_6, folate, vitamin B_{12}, zinc, vitamin C, and riboflavin. But the increase is not generally considered significant and therefore requires no special action—that is, if you eat a well-balanced diet. If your diet isn't the best, you should concentrate on achieving a more healthful diet, more for achieving overall good health than having anything to do with the use of oral contraceptives.

Menopause. After age 50, your need for iron decreases while calcium and vitamin D requirements increase. If you don't undergo hormone replacement therapy, which can protect against osteoporosis, it's especially important that you meet your needs for calcium and vitamin D—through food choices, supplements, or both. (see "Focus On...Calcium," page 22). Otherwise, no other significant changes in vitamin and mineral needs occur during or after menopause. There's no evidence that supplementation with any specific vitamin or mineral helps relieve symptoms of menopause such as mood swings and hot flashes. These appear to be more related to hormonal fluctuations.

Eating Habits and Other Choices

The choices you make in life, such as dieting to control weight, being a vegetarian, or smoking, can also affect your need for vitamin or mineral supplements.

Weight Control Diets. Cutting back on calories also means cutting back on nutrients, unless you're careful to make high-nutrient, low-calorie choices most of the time. The trouble is, because so many people are constantly "cutting back," they may become lax about food choices. It's easy to choose for taste or convenience over nutrition. And if you're cutting back severely, to less than 1200 calories a day, it may be almost impossible to meet all of your vitamin and mineral needs with food alone. While there is no substitute for healthy eating—especially when trying to control your weight—a multivitamin/mineral supplement with no more than 100 percent of the DV for vitamins and minerals may be a good idea if calorie concerns outweigh good intentions to eat nutritiously.

Poor Eating Habits. This situation can be the result of many things: not knowing what to eat for good health; hectic lifestyles that interfere with regular, well-balanced meals; poor appetite; or even just plain indifference about good nutrition. Whatever the reason, not eating recommended amounts of the five food groups on most days can lead to inadequate intakes of a variety of vitamins and minerals (as well as other important food components). If you're cutting out entire groups, you're certain to be missing out on essential nutrients.

Take a moment to assess your eating habits by comparing what you eat to the Food Guide Pyramid (page 15). If it adds up to poor nutrition, plan strategies to improve. A few simple changes might do the trick. Check with a registered dietitian if you can't come up with a plan by yourself. In the meantime, a multivitamin/mineral supplement with no more than 100 percent of the DV for vitamins and minerals might help fill a few nutrient gaps.

Vegetarian Diets. There are several types of vegetarian diets, classified according to what types of foods are excluded. Consisting primarily of plant foods, the lacto-vegetarian diet includes milk products whereas the lacto-ovovegetarian diet also includes eggs. Vegans, or total vegetarians, avoid all foods of animal origin.

All types of vegetarian diets can be healthy if they are appropriately planned. A vegetarian diet can also be based on the Food Guide Pyramid, with servings from the five food groups in recommended amounts—except for vegan diets. In this instance, the milk group is excluded.

This raises a question: Should vegans take calcium supplements, since dairy products are major sources of calcium? In fact, calcium deficiencies in any type of vegetarian diet are rare, and there is little evidence to show that calcium intakes below recommended levels cause major health problems in vegetarians. Studies show that vegetarians tend to absorb and retain more calcium from foods than do nonvegetarians. So the answer to the question is that vegans or other vegetarians do not appear to need calcium supplements.

Nor do they appear to need iron supplements. While they do

not consume heme iron, the form of iron in meats and poultry, vegetarians in general get greater amounts of vitamin C, which helps absorb non-heme iron from plant foods.

However, some vegans may need supplements of vitamin B_{12} in the form of cyanocobalamin (the form most readily absorbed in the body). Cyanocobalamin supplementation may be needed if you do not regularly eat a reliable source of the vitamin, such as fortified breakfast cereals, fortified soy beverages, and some brands of nutritional yeast. Spirulina, seaweed, tempeh, and other fermented foods are not reliable sources of vitamin B_{12}.

Children or adolescents who eat vegan diets should also have a reliable source of vitamin D. However, unless exposure to sunlight is limited, supplements are probably not needed. Calcium, iron, and zinc may also deserve special attention in children and adolescents, although intakes are usually adequate when a reasonable variety of food and adequate calories are eaten. Because vegetarian diets can be bulky, filling up a young child's small stomach quickly, take care that their diets supply enough calories to fuel their growth, development, and activities.

Pregnant and nursing vegetarians continue to need good sources of vitamin B_{12}. Like nonvegetarians, they are also frequently advised to take iron and folate (folic acid) supplements. A vitamin D supplement may be necessary if you spend little time in sunlight. Finally, you may need to pay special attention to eating foods rich in calcium.

Smoking. Research shows blood levels of vitamin C are lower in smokers than in nonsmokers. That means there's less vitamin C to tame free radicals—an important issue for smokers because smoke causes free radicals to form in the body (see "Focus on...Antioxidants," page 20). As a result, the RDA for vitamin C is higher for smokers—at least 100 milligrams daily compared to 60 milligrams per day for nonsmokers. But that amount is easily obtained from foods rich in vitamin C such as citrus fruits, peppers, cantaloupe, strawberries, broccoli, potatoes, kale, and cauliflower. Still, don't expect vitamin C to eliminate all the negative effects of smoking. Only stopping smoking can do that.

Along with research that has shown beta-carotene supplements provide little benefit to healthy people, two studies have observed an increased risk of cancer-related deaths in smokers taking beta-carotene supplements. In the second study, beta-carotene supplementation was discontinued to avoid any further possible harm to smoking participants.

Illness and Disease

Acquired Immune Deficiency Syndrome (AIDS). Purveyors of nutritional supplements such as vitamins, minerals, amino acids, and herbs may claim these substances protect against HIV infection, but experts agree that's only false hope. Once a person has the disease, however, it's a different story.

Because AIDS can seriously interfere with a person's ability to eat a well-balanced diet, as well as absorb and use nutrients, vitamin and mineral supplements are often a good idea. Active infections, the side effects of medications, lack of financial resources, depression, and brain dysfunction may all interfere with getting adequate nutrition. What's more, they may begin even in the early stages of this disease when no symptoms are present. And some researchers suggest that good nutritional health may be a primary factor in a person's ability to fight off progression from HIV infection to full-blown AIDS.

Be wary of large doses of supplements, however. They may carry the potential to do more harm than good. For example, 1000 or more milligrams of vitamin C can cause diarrhea, which can actually speed the progress of AIDS by further weakening the body and interfering with nutrient absorption.

Metabolic abnormalities may alter the significance of low blood values of vitamins and minerals, which may be used to judge nutritional status. That makes an individual nutritional assessment by a registered dietitian key to determining the most effective nutritional therapy for a person with AIDS.

Alzheimer's Disease. The cause of Alzheimer's disease is unknown, but there is no clear evidence that diet contributes to its development. The roles of certain vitamins in maintaining the health of the nervous system has led to the theory that large doses of these vitamins could help prevent or slow the progression of dementias of uncertain origin, such as Alzheimer's disease or other memory loss. But studies do not show patients with these problems improve as a result of megavitamin therapy.

Anemia. Anemia isn't a disease but instead a symptom of other health problems. With this condition, there aren't enough red blood cells, or hemoglobin in red blood cells, to transport oxygen to other body cells. The result is a lack of energy, often accompanied by pale skin, headache, weakness, lack of concentration, or irritability.

Iron deficiency is the most common cause of anemia, especially for women of child-bearing age and those who are pregnant (see "Focus on…Iron," page 24). But anemia may also result from problems such as a lack of vitamin B_{12} or folate, or other physical disorders. That makes it critical to find out the cause of the problem before attempting to solve it.

If a vitamin deficiency is the cause, it's important to know which one is lacking. People may become anemic because of a deficiency of folate or vitamin B_{12}. In the first case, getting enough folate can cure the problem. With vitamin B_{12} deficiency, however, folate may appear to take care of the anemia, but really only "covers up" the symptoms. It doesn't cure the other problems vitamin B_{12} deficiencies cause.

Some people lack intrinsic factor, a body chemical required to absorb vitamin B_{12}, and experience vitamin B_{12} deficiency. For these people, injections of vitamin B_{12} or high-dose oral supplements may be prescribed. Many older adults can no longer absorb adequate amounts of naturally-occurring vitamin B_{12} from foods and are advised to meet their needs for this vitamin by eating foods fortified with vitamin B_{12} and/or a vitamin B_{12}-containing supplement.

Bottom line: Consult your doctor if you suspect you are anemic, and follow his or her advice to remedy it.

Arthritis. Claims abound that special diets, foods, and supplements can help cure arthritis or even prevent it. But most claims are unproven. Many experts speculate the "placebo effect" may be at work when people report that a nutrient or other compound relieves their symptoms. In other words, it may be their belief in a treatment, not the treatment itself, that really provides the relief. The most scientifically-supported diet-related treatment for arthritis is to avoid excess weight and eat a well-balanced diet that fosters a healthy weight.

Experiments with fish oils have shown some positive results, but practical and safe doses are not known. Fish oil supplements may interfere with blood clotting and increase the risk of stroke, especially when taken with aspirin or other nonsteroidal anti-inflammatory drugs. They may also cause diarrhea and upset stomach. Getting the oil via fatty fish such as mackerel, salmon, sardines, or lake trout is the wiser course, at least until more is known about the safety and effectiveness of this therapy. Limited studies using a substance derived from cartilage, called glucosamine, have also shown some promise in relieving symptoms of osteoarthritis. However, as with other dietary supplements, the purity of glucosamine products sold in pharmacies, health food stores, and supermarkets is unknown.

Cancer. If you're taking vitamin or mineral supplements in high doses with the aim of preventing or treating cancer, especially lung and stomach cancer, consider this: So far, the best evidence supports the wisdom of eating a diet rich in whole grains, fruits, and vegetables (see "Focus on...Antioxidants," page 20) and low in fat to help prevent or slow the progress of cancer. Observational studies (see "Proving Cause & Effect," page 51) show such a diet does indeed appear to be linked to lower rates of many types of cancer.

So far, studies have not shown that supplements are effective in preventing cancer. More research is needed on the other components of whole grains, fruits, and vegetables. In the meantime, given that a diet rich in whole grains, fruits, and vegetables includes a host of food compounds that may fight cancer, the chances of seeing any real benefit are greater with food than with supplements, at least until science gives us a clearer answer.

If the effects of cancer do interfere with eating, check with a registered dietitian. He or she can advise you best whether vitamin and mineral supplements may be wise.

Carpal Tunnel Syndrome. Megadoses of vitamin B_6 are frequently recommended to relieve the symptoms of carpal tunnel syndrome (CTS), which include numbness, tingling, and pain in the hands and arms. But research indicates this therapy doesn't work. One double-blind study, in which neither the doctor nor the patient knew who got what treatment, showed those receiving 150 milligrams of vitamin B_6 (75 times the RDA) fared no better than those receiving a placebo. Another problem is that large doses of vitamin B_6 can cause nerve damage—exactly opposite the desired effect.

Chronic Fatigue Syndrome. Treatment with vitamins, amino acids, and magnesium supplements has been touted to help relieve the symptoms of chronic fatigue syndrome (CFS). But to date, it's neither known what causes the problem or what to do about it. The hallmark symptom is severe, disabling fatigue, sometimes accompanied by muscle weakness or pain, sleep problems, and trouble concentrating. If you do have CFS, eat a well-balanced diet. If you're often too tired to cook, stock up on quick and easy-to-prepare foods. Also consider supplementing your diet with oral supplements (see "Liquid [& Other] Nutrition," page 56).

Colds & Respiratory Illnesses. Although a popular theory, it's still not proven whether large doses of vitamin C will prevent colds. In controlled trials, vitamin C either did not reduce the frequency and severity of colds, or the effect was considerably smaller than originally reported. If you're eating a well-balanced diet, you're already getting enough vitamin C to help keep your immune system at its best. Indeed, average vitamin C intake in the United States is well above the RDA. Getting vitamin C from foods enhances your diet in other ways as well. More recently, zinc gluconate lozenges have been promoted to shorten the duration of a cold. Studies of its effectiveness are somewhat limited. We do know, however, that large amounts of zinc can be harmful, possibly impairing copper absorption, weakening immune response, and lowering levels of "good" (HDL) cholesterol.

Hair Loss. Hair loss may occur with an excess of vitamin A. Claims that you need extra vitamins such as biotin, pantothenic acid, B_6, C, and E as well as zinc to prevent hair loss haven't been substantiated.

One medication prescribed in the treatment of hair loss caused by hormonal abnormalities can increase the need for vitamin B_{12}. If you are undergoing such therapy, check with your physician about whether you need B_{12} supplements.

While on the subject of hair, it's also worthwhile to note that hair analyses are not reliable indicators of your nutritional health. The composition of hair depends on nutrients available in the diet, but it is also strongly affected by hair treatments. Shampoos, conditioners, and hair sprays, for example, can add or remove minerals from the hair.

Heart Disease. As with cancer, the benefit of any single vitamin or mineral in preventing or treating heart disease remains to be seen. Although vitamin E supplements have been associated with reduced heart disease risk in observational studies, such studies fail to prove cause and effect. An eight-year study with smokers found no effect of vitamin E on death rates. More studies are underway, but it's a matter of wait and see, and while we wait, making personal decisions. At this point, there is not enough information to justify everyone taking vitamin E supplements.

Recent research also points to the role of two B vitamins—folate (folic acid) and vitamin B_6—in protecting against heart disease. It seems these vitamins help clear the blood of the amino acid homocysteine, a byproduct of protein metabolism. High levels of homocysteine have been associated with an increased risk for heart attack and stroke. One study showed people with the lowest risk of heart attack had the highest intakes of folic acid and vitamin B_6—twice the RDA—providing even more reason to consume foods rich in these vitamins (see Appendix 1, page 79).

Large amounts of nicotinic acid, a form of the B vitamin niacin, have also been shown to reduce blood levels of low-density lipoproteins ("bad" cholesterol) while increasing levels of high-density lipoproteins ("good" cholesterol). But self-prescribed regimens can have serious side effects. Don't attempt the therapy on your own—see your doctor.

High Blood Pressure. Also known as hypertension, high blood pressure affects one in four Americans. For 95 percent of them, we don't know why. But a variety of factors may increase your risk for the disease, whether it "runs" in your family or if you're overweight, sedentary, or have diabetes. For men, risk increases after age 45 or so. For women, it goes up after menopause. Smoking and heavy drinking also add to your risk.

Up to 30 percent of Americans may be at risk for high blood pressure because of the amount of sodium they eat. These people are considered to have blood pressure that is "sodium-sensitive." Because there is no effective way to determine who is sodium sensitive and who is not, most people are advised to eat a diet moderate in salt and sodium (see Appendix 2, page 93).

Potassium, calcium, and magnesium also play a role in regulating blood pressure. Research shows a diet adequate in these minerals may help control high blood pressure. Eating the Food Guide Pyramid way—including plenty of whole grains, fruits, vegetables, and lower-fat dairy products—supplies necessary amounts of these minerals.

Osteoporosis. A lack of calcium, perhaps exacerbated by inadequate amounts of vitamin D, increases the risk for osteoporosis. But other factors are usually involved, too. See "Focus on...Calcium," page 22.

Stress. Physiological stress, such as that caused by surgery or other wounds (see below), may affect your nutritional needs. But the psychological stress many of us experience in our daily lives does not appear to increase our need for vitamins and minerals. In short, vitamin and mineral supplements can't relieve the ill effects of too much work or worry.

Surgery and Wound Healing. Good nutritional health before and after surgery helps heal wounds and decrease the risk of infections and other complications. It can also result in shorter hospital stays.

The stress of surgery increases protein losses in most patients, making this nutrient one of the most important to consider. Under normal conditions, a well-balanced diet can meet your needs adequately. But if your appetite is depressed before or after surgery, or if eating a well-balanced diet is otherwise interfered with, oral supplements may be a good idea (see "Liquid [& Other] Nutrition," page 56). Check with your doctor or registered dietitian first, however, to make certain other strategies are not necessary.

Oral supplements also contain a host of other vitamins and minerals that take part in the healing process. Among the most important are vitamin C and zinc, which help heal wounds. Extra iron may also be important if any blood loss occurred during the operation. If these nutrients are not obtained via dietary or oral supplements, other supplements may be called for. Check with your doctor or registered dietitian because too much of these micronutrients can cause problems, too.

Some surgical conditions require specific nutritional therapies that may include supplementation with vitamins and minerals. For example, stomach or intestinal surgery may interfere with normal digestion and absorption of vitamins and minerals. In such situations, vitamin/mineral supplements, as well as a controlled diet, are generally prescribed. Again, your doctor or registered dietitian should guide you in meeting your specific needs.

To "Optimize" Your Diet

While you may have heard that taking various types of supplements including vitamins and minerals can foster "optimal" health, there's little evidence at this point for such claims.

The best nutritional approach is to get your nutrients from food, primarily because scientists have not yet determined everything there is in food that contributes to health. Nor do we know the precise amounts we need of many food compounds we have identified. It's also unclear how the many food compounds all work together, or how a higher intake of one might affect absorption or use of another.

In short, foods contain a "package" of substances, in a unique mix, essential to health. The best advice at this point is to first choose the recommended amounts of different foods to foster optimal health.

If you do opt for supplements along with a balanced diet, choose those that contain no more than 100 percent of the Daily Value for vitamins and minerals. That way, you'll reduce chances of getting too much of any one vitamin or mineral, which may cause harm or interfere with other vitamins and minerals. And be wary of supplements about which we know little, or which we do know can be harmful. Review "Dietary Supplements—Separating Fact from Fancy" on page 65.

Do Medicines Affect Your Vitamin and Mineral Needs?*

Before taking any medication, whether prescribed or over-the-counter, ask your pharmacist about drug-food interactions associated with it. For example, you may be advised to take the medication before, after, or with meals. Or you may be told to avoid certain foods or alcohol when taking the drug.

Many factors may need to be considered when taking medications, and you should depend on your doctor or pharmacist to guide you in their effective use.

The following information covers the interaction of certain medications with specific vitamins and minerals. It is not intended to be a comprehensive guide or replace your physician's or pharmacist's advice.

To Treat Acne: Isotretinoin (Accutane)—Do not take supplements containing vitamin A.

To Thin Blood/Anticoagulant: Warfarin (Coumadin, Panwarfarin)—Do not suddenly eat more foods high in vitamin K than usual. Do not take any supplements that contain vitamin E or vitamin K. Do not drink herbal teas containing coumarin.

To Lower Blood Cholesterol: Cholestyramine (Questran, Cholybar), Colestipol (Colestid)—Used over an extended period may deplete body stores of vitamins A, D, E, and K, beta carotene, and folate. Ask doctor or registered dietitian whether supplements are needed.

To Treat High Blood Pressure or Heart Conditions: Angiotensin-Converting Enzyme (ACE) Inhibitors—Benazepril (Lotensin), Captopril (Capoten), Enalapril (Vasotec), Quinapril (Accupril)—May need to limit sodium and salt. Do not take potassium supplements or use salt substitutes that contain potassium.

Loop Diuretics—Furosemide (Lasix), Bumetanide (Bumex),

---

*Adapted from *Patient Education Materials: A Supplement to Handbook on Drug and Nutrient Interactions*, Fifth Edition, by Daphne A. Roe, MD, The American Dietetic Association, Chicago, IL, 1994.

Ethacrynic acid (Edecrin)—May deplete potassium and thiamin. Eat high-potassium and thiamin-containing foods daily unless your doctor has told you not to. May need to limit sodium and salt.

Thiazide Diuretics—Chlorothiazide (Diuril), Hydrochlorothiazide (Esidrix, HydroDIURIL, Oretic)—May deplete potassium. Eat high-potassium foods daily unless your doctor has told you not to. May need to limit sodium and salt.

Miscellaneous—Digoxin (Lanoxin)—Prevent appetite changes that cause weight loss by eating high-potassium foods daily. Take 1 hour before breakfast, and avoid high-fiber foods or supplements at that meal.

Hydralazine (Apresoline)—May need to limit sodium and salt.

To Treat Crohn's Disease, Colitis, or Other Bowel Conditions: Sulfasalazine (Azulfidine)—May cause anemia due to lack of folate. Doctor may recommend supplement, or foods high in folate daily.

To Treat Infections: Tetracycline (Achromycin V, Panmycin, Robitet, Sumycin), Oxytetracycline (Terramycin)—Avoid the following foods, supplements, and medicines for at least 1 hour before and after each dose: milk, yogurt, cheese, other dairy products, calcium supplements, iron supplements, antacids, magnesium-containing laxatives.

To Relieve Pain: Nonsteroidal Anti-inflammatory Drugs— Diclofenac (Voltaren), Diflunisal (Dolobid), Ibuprofen (Advil, Motrin), Indomethacin (Indocin), Naproxen (Naprosyn, Anaprox), Piroxicam (Feldene), Sulinac (Clinoril), Tolmetin (Tolectin)—Increase risk of gastrointestinal blood loss. Eat iron-rich foods daily. May need to limit sodium and salt.

To Treat Parkinson's Disease: Levodopa (Dopar)—Do not take with high-protein foods or supplements.

To Treat Seizure Disorders: Phenytoin (Dilantin)—Can cause folate deficiency; eat at least 1 serving of green vegetables daily. Intake of more than 5 mg of folate daily can interfere with seizure control. Drink 2 to 3 glasses of milk daily to prevent bone disease.

To Treat Tuberculosis: Isoniazid (Nydrazid)—Physician may recommend vitamin B_6 and vitamin D supplements.

Proving Cause & Effect—Interpreting Study Results

All studies are not created equal. Observational studies, in which researchers observe what people eat and the subsequent rates of disease, only point out potential relationships between diet and disease. To find out if the development of a disease truly is affected by what is eaten, intervention trials must be conducted in which people follow specific test diets.

Still, observational studies can provide important guidance. Most of the research connecting a diet rich in grains, fruits, and vegetables with a reduced risk of chronic disease is observational. But because such a diet poses few risks and offers substantial benefits, nutrition experts agree it's a wise strategy for promoting health.

The bottom line: Carefully consider how a study is conducted, look for other studies that confirm the findings, and put all findings in context of the total diet. If you're more confused than informed by what you hear and read, check with a registered dietitian who can help you translate research findings into straightforward guidelines for promoting health through diet.

As you can see, the question of whether a vitamin/mineral supplement would be beneficial for you depends on many circumstances. Your age, sex, eating habits, health, and other factors can impact the decision to take a vitamin/mineral supplement. But which supplement is best? Chapter 4 will lead the way.

Chapter Four

Choosing a Supplement

WITH SO MANY vitamin and mineral supplement choices on store shelves, choosing the right one can be a real challenge. Should you take more than the Daily Value (DV)? Are "natural" vitamins any better than synthetic ones? Can you trust the claims on the labels? Read on for answers to these and more questions.

How Much Is Enough?

While more may be better when it comes to many things, that old axiom just doesn't hold true in the case of vitamins and minerals. Consumed in excessive amounts over a long period, some supplements may do more harm than good. Undesirable effects range from fatigue, diarrhea, and hair loss to more serious problems such as kidney stones, liver or nerve damage, birth defects, and even death.

For example, vitamins A and D have long been known to be toxic, or poisonous, when taken in excess over an extended time. Too much vitamin A in the body can lead to bone and liver damage, headaches, diarrhea, and birth defects. Too much vitamin D causes kidney damage and bone deformity. Bottom line: Either as single or combination vitamin or mineral supplements, taking too much can be dangerous.

Low levels of single vitamin or mineral supplements may cause problems, too. Imbalances of vitamins or minerals can occur due to the effect of one nutrient on another. For example, zinc supplements can interfere with copper absorption, potentially creating a deficiency of copper.

Your best bet: If your situation calls for supplements, choose those that offer no more than 100 percent of the Daily Value (DV) for vitamins and minerals, unless you are otherwise advised by your doctor or registered dietitian.

Remember, too, that supplements are no substitute for a healthful eating plan. Indeed, many nutrition experts worry that people who take vitamin/mineral pills live with a false sense of security. They could wrongly assume that the pills make it less critical to pay attention to what they eat. But a healthy lifestyle that includes a well-balanced diet remains the primary strategy for getting and staying healthy.

Choosing the Right Supplement

If you decide, or have been advised, to take a supplement, these tips can help.

> ➤ Look for a combination of vitamins and minerals—in amounts that don't exceed 100 percent of the DV. However, don't expect to get 100 percent of nutrients such as calcium and magnesium. They're too bulky to fit into one tablet. Avoid large doses of any nutrient, unless recommended by your doctor or registered dietitian.

> ➤ Choose a supplement that meets your unique needs. Age, sex, and medical status are factors to consider. But don't just go by the label claim. Compare the vitamins and minerals the supplement offers against your particular needs. Don't be taken in by preparations that claim to have an effect that science doesn't support, such as supplements to help stop hair loss. See "Label Smarts: What Can You Trust?", on page 55. Also, if your needs can be met by a standard supplement, you don't need to spend the extra money a special preparation may cost.

> ➤ Don't be lured by extra ingredients that offer no proven benefits, such as inositol, lecithin, and PABA.

> ➤ Choose a supplement that's easy to swallow. Calcium supplements, for example, can be large and difficult to take. Some supplements are coated for easier swallowing.

➤ To save money, consider the generic or store brand. Brand name preparations usually offer no advantage—they just cost more! (See "Getting What You Pay For" on page 60.)

➤ Check the expiration date on the label. Over time, some vitamins lose their potency.

Once you buy dietary supplements, there are new responsibilities. Keep these guidelines in mind, too:

➤ Buy supplements in childproof containers, then store them in a safe place, away from the reach of children. More children die in the United States each year from accidental poisoning with adult iron supplements than any other substance.

➤ During regular medical check-ups, remind your physician about any dietary supplements you take. And if you're taking medications, be sure to talk with your doctor. Supplements can block the action of some medications (see "Do Medicines Affect Your Vitamin and Mineral Needs?", on page 49).

➤ Remember, food before pills. Supplements can only complement, not replace, a healthy diet. Also, if you skip a meal, you don't need to double dose. Make up your missed meal with wise food choices when you eat again.

Label Smarts: What Can You Trust?

Have any labels of dietary supplements made you sit up and take notice? Phrases such as "makes wrinkles disappear," "improves sexual response," and "prevents cancer," will catch anyone's eye. But can you believe what you read?

The answer is no and yes. For decades, the Food and Drug Administration (FDA) regulated dietary supplements as foods to ensure they were safe and wholesome and that their labeling was truthful. A component of ensuring safety was FDA's evaluation of the safety of all new ingredients, including those used in dietary supplements. However, with passage of the Dietary Supplement Health and Education Act (DSHEA) of 1994, provisions that apply only to dietary supplements and their ingredients were created. (Remember, dietary supplements can be any product that contains one or more dietary ingredients such as vitamins, minerals, herbs or other botanicals, amino acids, enzymes, extracts, or other ingredients used to supplement the diet.) As a result of these provisions, dietary ingredients used in dietary supplements are no longer subject to premarket safety evaluations required of other new food ingredients.

Why this seemingly "hands-off" policy? In part, this change was due to the millions of responses from consumers and manufacturers to the initial proposals to better regulate supplement claims. It boils down to the fact that consumers want dietary supplements to be available without prescriptions and manufacturers want to be able to sell supplements with minimal regulation. In addition, the FDA already has limited resources to analyze the composition of food products, let alone dietary supplements. So the responsibility now rests with manufacturers who must ensure that the ingredient list is accurate, the ingredients are safe, and that the content matches the amounts declared on the label. Keep in mind—this means that manufacturers and distributors do not need to register with the FDA or get FDA approval before producing or selling dietary supplements.

Liquid (& Other) Nutrition

If you are having trouble eating because of illness, lack of appetite, or chewing or swallowing difficulties, oral supplements can provide important nutrition. Not intended to replace food, these supplements can help "fill the gaps" with energy, protein, carbohydrates, fat, vitamins, minerals, and, in some cases, fiber to complement meals and snacks.

Oral supplements come in a range of textures, temperatures, colors, and shapes in the form of beverages, thick shakes, fruit juices, chewy bars, smooth puddings, savory soups, crunchy cookies—even hot decaffeinated coffees.

People with special nutritional requirements may also find oral supplements designed for them. Examples include supplements with extra calories or protein for people who need to gain weight or promote wound healing, those just for children recovering from illness, or choices for people who have HIV/AIDS or stomach or gastrointestinal problems.

Supplement Facts

Serving Size 1 Tablet

	Amount Per Serving	% Daily Value
Vitamin A (as retinyl acetate and 50% as beta-carotene)	5000 IU	100%
Vitamin C (as ascorbic acid)	60 mg	100%
Vitamin D (as cholecalciferol)	400 IU	100%
Vitamin E (as d-alpha tocopheryl acetate)	30 IU	100%
Thiamin (as thiamin mononitrate)	1.5 mg	100%
Riboflavin	1.7 mg	100%
Niacin (as niacinamide)	20 mg	100%
Vitamin B_6 (as pyridoxine hydrochloride)	2.0 mg	100%
Folate (as folic acid)	400 mcg	100%
Vitamin B_{12} (as cyanocobalamin)	6 mcg	100%
Biotin	30 mcg	10%
Pantothenic Acid (as calcium pantothenate)	10 mg	100%

Other ingredients: Gelatin, lactose, magnesium stearate, microcrystalline cellulose, FD&C Yellow No. 6, propylene glycol, propylparaben, and sodium benzoate.

Dietary supplements are required to carry a Supplement Facts panel (above), similar to the Nutrition Facts panel on food products. To be a savvy supplement shopper, it's important to understand what can and cannot be stated on supplement labels.

Information that *must* be provided on supplement labels:
- ➤Appropriate serving size (determined by manufacturer)
- ➤Amounts and % DV (per serving stated) for 14 nutrients, if present at significant levels, including sodium, vitamin A, vitamin C, calcium, and iron, and other vitamins and minerals if they are added or are part of a nutritional claim.
- ➤Names and amounts of other dietary ingredients for which no DVs have been established. If a proprietary blend of ingredients is contained in a supplement, only the names of the ingredients and the total amount of the blend must be listed.
- ➤A complete list of ingredients in decreasing order by weight. If an ingredient is listed in the nutrition labeling,

Choosing a Supplement

such as "calcium from calcium gluconate," it need not appear in the list of ingredients.

Other information *allowed* on supplement labels:

➤The term "high potency" can be used if the supplement contains 100 percent or more of the established DV for that vitamin or mineral; or with multi-ingredient products, if two-thirds of the nutrients are present at levels more than 100 percent of the DV.

➤The term "antioxidant" may be used to describe a supplement that contains nutrients, such as vitamin C, in an amount sufficient and known to inactivate harmful free radicals in the body.

➤Statements of nutritional support that give the manufacturer's description of the effects of the dietary supplement on the *structure* or *functioning* of the body are permitted on labels. Examples include "promotes regularity" or "supports the immune system." But because the statements are not authorized by the FDA, you'll see the following disclaimer on labels that make nutrition claims: "This statement has not been evaluated by the FDA. This product is not intended to diagnose, treat, cure, or prevent any disease."

➤Only FDA-approved health claims, which describe the connection between a nutrient or food substance and a disease or health-related condition, can be included if the content of the product meets the established FDA requirements.

Information that *cannot* be included on supplement labels:

➤Statements that claim a dietary supplement can treat, diagnose, cure, or prevent a disease are not allowed. Examples include "protects against cancer," "treats hot flashes," and "reduces nausea associated with chemotherapy."

➤Nutrition and health claims that are false or misleading are also prohibited, but this doesn't mean you won't encounter some claims that seem to fit in this category.

Sensible advice is to forget some of the more provocative claims you see. If they sound too good to be true, they probably are.

The bottom line: It's still up to you to be an informed consumer. Even though labeling of dietary supplements is now more uniform and easier to read, the safety or effectiveness of a dietary supplement in the dosage provided isn't regulated. Investigate the benefits—and risks—before you take any kind of dietary supplement.

Supplement Savvy

Does it makes a difference when you take a vitamin or mineral supplement? In general, it's a good idea to take it with meals. That's because some vitamins and minerals are better absorbed when taken with food. Most iron supplements are better absorbed when taken *between* meals, however. And if you take calcium and iron, take them at separate times. Calcium can interfere with iron absorption.

Do time-release preparations offer any advantages? Not likely. In fact, the coatings used to control the release may interfere with the absorption of fat-soluble vitamins. What's more, some evidence indicates that time-release niacin formulations could harm the liver. One exception: Time-released iron supplements may be less likely than regular preparations to upset your stomach.

Are chelated or esterified supplements better than standard varieties? These are just marketing gimmicks. If you want assurance that you're getting vitamins and minerals in their most usable form for the body, look instead for "USP" on the label. That means the product meets standards set by the U.S. Pharmacopeia for purity, potency, and availability. See "Getting What You Pay For" on page 60 for more on standards of quality.

Are stress formulas necessary? Physical stress, such as surgery or other injuries, may increase the need for some nutrients (see "Surgery and Wound Healing," page 47). But the stress from busy, harried, or worry-filled lives doesn't affect our nutritional needs. If such stress is getting you down, you'd do better to adopt proven stress reduction methods such as regular exercise and relaxation techniques.

Are supplements from "natural" sources better than synthetic versions?
Usually, there's no need to spend the extra money for "natural" preparations. Sometimes it may even be to your disadvantage. For example, synthetic folate is more easily absorbed. And calcium supplements with dolomite, oyster shell, or bone meal can contain small amounts of lead and other undesirable metals. However, for vitamin E, the natural form does appear to be retained by the body better than the synthetic form. For some nutrients, you may need to take more tablets of "natural" preparations to get the same amount found in other synthetic supplements. In some instances, vitamins labeled "natural" may actually be mixtures of natural and synthetic forms.

Do vitamins or other supplements such as bee pollen and spirulina boost your energy? Some vitamins, such as thiamin, do play a role in energy production. But taking more than you need isn't going to give you more energy. Only food—or the carbohydrates, fat, protein, and alcohol in it—provides energy. Substances such as bee pollen or spirulina don't offer any magical benefits in this or any other regard, either.

Can supplements help detoxify your body? Your body has its own detoxification system: the liver and kidneys. They break down toxic byproducts in the body, and don't need any outside help in healthy people. Nor is there any proof that supplements of any kind can help, whether you're healthy or not. In the case of kidney failure, the only way to remove toxic byproducts is through dialysis, which removes blood from the body to be filtered.

··

Getting What You Pay For

Consider this: Are the vitamins and minerals in the supplement you're thinking about taking absorbed into your body where they're needed? Until recently, there's been no guarantee that a supplement would break down in the stomach to release vitamins and minerals for absorption! That prompted the U.S. Pharmacopeia (USP), the organization that sets federal standards for drugs and supplements, to

Vitamins, Minerals, and Dietary Supplements

establish quality standards. They include the time a supplement takes to disintegrate and dissolve.

When purchasing supplements, look for "USP" on the label. This means that the supplement meets strict standards for dissolution, disintegration, strength, and purity. Some manufacturers give their own assurance with the words "proven release," "laboratory tested," "quality and potency guaranteed," or something similar, but there's no legal meaning for these phrases. Many supplements don't list any such guarantees. If the brand you prefer doesn't have "USP" on the label, call the company to find out if the product passed a one-hour dissolution test.

Chapter Five
Dietary Supplements and Other Products

YOU NOW KNOW that, in most cases, extra vitamins and minerals aren't necessary if you're eating healthfully. But what about all the other types of supplements: herbs, amino acids, fish oil, blue-green algae, shark cartilage...the list goes on. Should you seriously consider adding any of these to your daily regimen for good health?

The best place to start is with some general guidelines for judging whether supplement claims (or for that matter, any claims about food and nutrition) are true. Look for these warning signals that a claim has no basis in science. They come from the Food and Nutrition Alliance, a group of four nutrition organizations including The American Dietetic Association.

How to spot "junk science."

➤ It promises a quick fix.

➤ It sounds too good to be true.

➤ It makes a simple conclusion based on the findings of a complex study.

➤ It makes recommendations based on a single study.

➤ Recommendations are made based on studies published without peer review. If you can't judge the quality of a published study, check with your doctor or a registered dietitian.

➤ The recommendations are made to sell a product. This may apply particularly to advice you receive from a salesperson.

➤ The recommendations come from studies that ignore differences among individuals and groups.

➤ Dramatic statements about the effectiveness of the supplement are refuted by reputable scientific organizations.

Also, if the claim is based on testimonials from satisfied customers, you're wise to look further. Unless scientific studies back them up, benefits based on individual reports may be more due to the placebo effect than anything else. That is, the benefit or improvement in a situation can be due to a person's belief that a treatment works; but when scientifically tested, the treatment doesn't prove to be effective.

While the placebo effect may seem beneficial in the case of less serious ailments such as headaches, be aware of the risks you take. At the least, many people waste their money by succumbing to unproven claims for supplements. But the danger can be much greater than that. People have died from taking some types of dietary supplements. Others have postponed conventional treatment for serious diseases, opting instead for therapies that offer no real benefit.

One other caveat: Minimal regulation in the dietary supplement industry makes it almost impossible to know if supplements contain what they say they do, and if there's anything there that shouldn't be. Further, there may be little research to back up claims. As a result, in many cases, no one knows the safe dosage and long-term effects of taking some dietary supplements.

If you still want to try a dietary supplement, don't make the decision without first checking with a reputable source; your doctor, registered dietitian, or pharmacist is a good start. They will at least be able to tell you if there is any evidence of harm associated with taking the supplement. They can also explore your personal situation to determine if there are any reasons you shouldn't use the supplement. And they may be able to tell you if any evidence exists that a supplement can do what its manufacturers claim. In general, however, most dietary supplements are not recommended for use by pregnant or nursing women or children.

Here's what we can tell you about some of the dietary supplements you'll find in stores today. The following information helps you separate the facts from the fantasies about whether these substances can play a role in guarding or promoting your good health. It also warns you of some potentially harmful substances you should avoid.

The information about the dietary supplements cited in the following list is included to give you insight into the true potential of these substances. While the information presented here is based on current research and knowledge, scientists are just beginning to learn about the potential benefits and risks of many dietary supplements.

Dietary Supplements—Separating Fact from Fancy

Aloe vera juice (an herbal product)

The claims—Gentle laxative. One company promotes it as a "catalyst" to make its other herbal supplements work faster.

The facts—There's no proof of the second claim, but it is known that aloe vera taken internally does act as a laxative. Trouble is, the effects aren't necessarily gentle.

Amino Acids & Protein Supplements

The claims—A remedy for obesity, insomnia, depression, pain, and infections. Most frequent claim: Builds muscles.

The facts—We get plenty in our diets, and even make some amino acids in our bodies. But they offer no special benefits in the body beyond serving as protein "building blocks." In fact, excess amino acids are simply used for energy, and may be converted to body fat if you exceed your energy needs. High doses of one amino acid can also decrease absorption and utilization of others. A few years ago, contaminated batches of L-tryptophan, an amino acid promoted to aid sleep, killed 38 people and caused permanent neurological damage in hundreds more.

Bee pollen

The claims—Nature's most perfect food, with benefits ranging from boosting energy to curing impotence, and everything in between.

The facts—Contains starch, sugars, protein, a small amount

of fat, and perhaps some vitamins—the same nutrients found naturally in food with the same benefits and nothing more. Some people may experience allergic reactions to bee pollen.

Blue-green algae (an herbal product, also known as spirulina)

The claims—A "superfood" that helps control appetite, boost energy and immunity, and detoxify the body, while helping to treat diseases ranging from Alzheimer's to jet lag.

The facts—The only claim science backs up is that it contains protein, beta carotene, and small amounts of minerals such as zinc. At the high price spirulina goes for, we can get these nutrients in much more economical forms.

Bioflavonoids (hesperidin, rutin, quercetin, vitamin P)

The claims—Relieves pain, promotes circulation, lowers cholesterol, and treats and prevents cataracts and asthma.

The facts—The relationship between flavonoids and chronic disease is under study, but at present, it is not known whether they have any nutritional effect. They are also found in generous amounts in citrus fruits and other fruits and vegetables.

Carnitine

The claims—Helps burn body fat and improve athletic endurance.

The facts—While it is a necessary substance, research indicates the body produces enough, and supplements don't help. Deficiencies are only seen in people with severe malabsorption problems, those on dialysis, people who are fed parenterally (through the veins), or those who have a genetic carnitine deficiency. Even then, supplements don't necessarily cure the problem.

Chaparral (an herbal product)

The claims—Purifies blood, cures cancer, treats acne, and is a natural antioxidant. Improves kidney, lung, and liver function.

The facts—Rather than improving liver function, it has reportedly caused severe liver damage in some people. Other claims not substantiated. Not recommended.

Chromium picolinate

The claims—Aids weight loss, builds muscle, reduces blood sugar and cholesterol, and prevents osteoporosis.

The facts—Chromium is a "cofactor" for insulin, which means it does play a role in maintaining normal blood sugar. But dietary-induced deficiencies of chromium are extremely rare. What's more, researchers report there's no evidence for claims about chromium picolinate, and warn of possible health risks, particularly in the large amounts many athletes take. Even single doses of many preparations contain much more than the RDA for chromium.

Coenzyme Q10 (also known as ubiquinone)

The claims—Prevents heart disease and aging, boosts immunity, aids weight loss, and cures gum disease.

The facts—Made by the body, it may act as an antioxidant. There's no evidence we need to get it from the diet, and experts disagree whether it's even effective when taken by mouth. Other reports say it works like a drug and carries harmful side effects, so medical supervision is required with use.

Comfrey (an herbal product)

The claims—Heals wounds, cleans wounds, and treats asthma, coughs, ulcers, cramps, tuberculosis, pain, and burns.

The facts—The oral use of any comfrey product is strongly discouraged. Comfrey has caused severe liver damage and can be extremely harmful if you use it while taking any other medication.

Echinacea (an herbal product)

The claims—Boosts immunity, especially for upper respiratory infections (colds).

The facts—Research suggests it can increase resistance to upper respiratory infections, but continued use longer than 6 to 8 weeks may decrease resistance. People allergic to the sunflower family may have reactions.

Enzymes

The claims—Aids digestion.

The facts—Our bodies generally make the enzymes we need, except in rare cases of "inborn errors of metabolism." Common exceptions: People who cannot tolerate milk may lack the enzyme lactase. Lactase-treated milk, or lactase supplements taken with dairy foods, can improve the problem. Some enzymes can also help reduce gas production from legumes. Saliva and stomach acid production may decrease with age, but there's no evidence we don't make enough enzymes to adequately digest food. Most metabolic enzymes taken as supplements are broken down into component parts before absorption, destroying enzymatic activity.

Ephedra (an herbal product, also known as ephedrine, pseudo-ephrine, ma huang, epitonin)

The claims—Controls weight and boosts energy.

The facts—The dangers far outweigh potential benefits. Risks include: high blood pressure, palpitations, nerve damage, muscle injury, psychosis, stroke, and memory loss. Linked to about a dozen deaths so far.

Fat burners

The claims—Aids weight loss.

The facts—Unfortunately, the only way to burn fat is to use more energy than you take in. Translation: Eat less, exercise more!

Feverfew (an herbal product)

The claims—Treats headaches, especially migraines; relieves arthritis, indigestion, colds, fever, and muscle tension; stimulates appetite.

The facts—Only documented benefit: May work for migraine relief. May also cause mouth ulcers.

Fiber supplements

The claims—Works as a laxative and aids weight control.

The facts—Increasing fiber is proven to aid regularity. A fiber-rich diet may be lower in fat and calories, too, helping weight control. High-fiber foods are preferred because they contain a variety of fibers that may play beneficial roles in health. If you take supplements, do not exceed 35 grams of fiber per day (including the fiber you get from food). Drink plenty of fluids to avoid intestinal obstructions. Increase fiber from food or supplements slowly to avoid problems with cramping, diarrhea, and flatulence.

Fish oil

The claims—Protects against heart disease, cancer, and arthritis.

The facts—It's controversial whether omega-3 fatty acids found in fish oils offer such benefits. But experts agree eating fish several times a week is the best way to get the benefits, if they do exist, without risks such as excessive bleeding, drug interactions, or even high cholesterol. Try salmon, mackerel, sardines, herring, whitefish, oyster, shark, smelt, squid, swordfish, and pompano.

Garlic

The claims—Reduces blood cholesterol levels and prevents cancer.

The facts—There is some indication garlic reduces blood cholesterol and triglycerides. Large doses may cause stomach irritation or nausea. Real garlic is the most reliable source of active ingredients, but eating the one to four raw cloves required daily to produce effects may result in bad breath. If you take anticoagulant medications, use garlic supplements only on your physician's advice. Garlic cannot substitute for a prescribed medical regimen for those with heart disease, nor for a healthy lifestyle and eating plan for those who don't have the disease.

Ginger (an herbal product)

The claims—Reduces motion sickness and other nausea.

The facts—Taken before traveling and as symptoms begin to occur, this herb may help prevent the nausea of motion sickness. Check with a pharmacist whether you should try it, and, if so, how much you need.

Ginkgo biloba (an herbal product)

The claims—Treats circulatory disorders, asthma, and Alzheimer's; reverses aging; increases mental performance, memory, and concentration; and reduces tension.

The facts—Studies show it may enhance blood flow to the brain, which may have some effect on symptoms such as dizziness, depression, tinnitus, and short-term memory loss. May also aid circulation in legs and relieve cramps. Other claims are not substantiated. Side effects include gastrointestinal disturbance, headaches, and allergic skin reactions.

Gingseng (an herbal product)

The claims—You name it, it cures it! Also a tonic, "restorative," aphrodisiac, and life extender.

The facts—Studies indicate the placebo effect is probably at work with gingseng users. But experts agree long-term, carefully controlled studies are needed. Another obstacle: Supplements vary widely in their content of the supposed active ingredient "ginsenosides."

Inositol

The claims—Treats baldness, lowers blood cholesterol, and aids weight control.

The facts—If mice eating highly-purified diets don't get enough, they lose hair, but humans don't suffer similarly. Further, your diet contains plenty—and your body manufactures plenty, too.

Jin bu huan (an herbal product)

The claims—Aids sleep and relieves back pain.

The facts—May provide reported benefits, but risks are high: People taking the supplement as directed contracted hepatitis. Best bet: Ask your doctor for sleep aids or pain relievers that have been tested for effectiveness and safety.

Kombucha tea (an herbal product, also known as mushroom tea, Japanese tea fungus, kargasok, manchurian, kvass tea, teakwass, kwassan)

The claims—Cures AIDS, cancer, and psoriasis; burns body fat; detoxifies the body; enhances memory; dissolves kidney stones—the list goes on and on.

The facts—Benefits aren't proven. Reportedly has caused liver and other organ damage, gastrointestinal upset, and death. May also interfere with medications, and has potential to cause allergic reactions. Good advice: Avoid it!

Lecithin

The claims—Lowers blood cholesterol; improves memory; cures arthritis, high blood pressure, and gallbladder problems; and controls weight.

The facts—Studies show no benefit for supplements. Memory claims are based on the fact that it contains choline (see "Choline," page 91).

Lobelia (an herbal product)

The claims—Suppresses cough, reduces fever and cold symptoms, and treats sore throats, laryngitis, colic, asthma, bronchitis, angina, and epilepsy.

The facts—Low doses may act as a nicotine-like stimulant to dilate lung bronchi and aid breathing. Reported negative effects include decreased blood pressure, sweating, coma, and death from larger doses. Check with your doctor or pharmacist for safer aids.

Melatonin

The claims—Aids sleep, fights jet lag, lowers blood cholesterol, prevents breast cancer, aids birth control, and treats Alzheimer's, Parkinson's, and cataracts.

The facts—Supplements may aid sleep for people who are deficient in this hormone produced by a gland in the brain. Other benefits or effects in healthy normal people are still under investigation. Likewise, the possible side effects of long-term supplementation with melatonin are unknown. Use only with doctor's supervision. The following people should avoid it completely: people on steroid medications, women who want to become or who already are pregnant or nursing, the mentally ill, people with severe allergies, those with autoimmune diseases or cancers of the immune system, and children.

PABA (paraminobenzoic acid)

The claims—Protects against sunburn and skin cancer; helps utilize protein and make red blood cells; restores gray hair to natural color.

The facts—This "growth factor" is made in the body; we don't need any from food or supplements. No benefits have been shown except when used externally for sunburn protection.

Pectin

The claims—Controls blood sugar in people with diabetes, detoxifies blood, and lowers cholesterol.

The facts—As a soluble fiber, it may help control blood sugar levels and lower blood cholesterol. But you can get plenty in foods such as apples, citrus fruits, carrots, and bananas. Other foods high in soluble fiber include oats and beans.

Phytochemicals

The claims—Helps prevent cancer, heart disease, and a host of other diseases afflicting us as we grow older.

The facts—Science points to a role for phytochemicals (biologically active chemicals in plants) in protecting against disease. But experts recommend food, particularly whole grains, fruits, and vegetables, over supplements—we haven't yet identified all of the phytochemicals, nor do we know how they work together. What's more, the potential risks of phytochemical supplements haven't been explored.

Saw palmetto (an herbal product)

The claims—Treats enlarged prostate.

The facts—May improve urinary flow in men with non-cancerous enlarged prostates. Should not substitute for proper medical treatment. Use only with doctor's supervision. Teas made from the substance are not effective.

Shark cartilage (also known as glucosamine)

The claims—Reduces muscle stiffness and treats inflamed joints. Reduces the risk for and treats cancer.

The facts—Sharks do get cancer, even though some may claim otherwise. What's more, studies don't show shark cartilage works as cancer treatment. Glucosamine might hold some promise for treating osteoarthritis, but most studies have been short, with unconvincing results.

St. John's wort (an herbal product)

The claims—Alleviates depression, anxiety, and sleep disturbances.

The facts—Appears to be moderately effective in treating mild depression. May be prescribed as an alternative to drug therapy. Taking this herb may make your skin more sensitive to the sun.

Valerian root (an herbal product)

The claims—Aids sleep, treats nervousness, ulcers, headaches, pain, convulsions, and muscle cramps, and improves circulation.

The facts—May have a sedative, tranquilizing effect. This herb was once listed as an official drug, but according to one expert, lost that status not because it was ineffective, but because it could not compete with more widely-used drugs. Side effects have not been reported.

Weight gain supplements
The claims—Helps add pounds.

The facts—Weight gain supplements offer no more benefits than a well-balanced diet that contains plenty of calories. But actual foods don't cost as much, and probably taste a lot better. Check with a registered dietitian if you can't gain wanted pounds; you'll get a plan that provides for good health, too.

Yohimbe (an herbal product)
The claims—Aphrodisiac

The facts—The active ingredient, yohimbine, is a drug prescribed to treat impotence, but appears to be ineffective. Reported effects of too much yohimbe include paralysis, fatigue, stomach problems, and death.

Chapter Six
The Last Word

WITH SO MUCH INTEREST in the potential protective health effects of vitamins, minerals, and other substances in the diet, researchers worldwide are devoting their careers to studying these compounds. That means you'll continue to see headlines heralding new discoveries about the benefits—or harmful consequences—of substances ranging from antioxidants to phytochemicals to ingredients we haven't even heard of yet. How do you begin to make sense of the headlines, particularly when they seem to conflict from one day to the next?

Reading Between the Lines

Here are some quick tips for ferreting out the real facts in nutrition reports as well as in advertisements for nutritional products.

➤ Be wary if immediate, effortless, or guaranteed results are promised. Watch out, too, for telltale words and phrases such as "breakthrough," "miracle," "secret remedy," "exclusive," and "clinical studies prove that…" It's rare that any of these claims prove true. And if it sounds too good to be true, it probably is!

➤ Don't accept one report as the final word. Reporters and editors face deadlines and space and time limitations that often get in the way of telling the whole story.

➤ Don't take action based on a single study. Scientists usually don't put their faith in research results until they have been duplicated by other scientists.

➤ Look beyond the headlines to investigate the type of study that reported the results. Was it an observational study (see "Proving Cause & Effect," page 51)? Or was it a well-controlled intervention study that truly tested the effects of a type of diet or substance?

➤ Ask how you compare to whom or what is studied before you make any dietary changes. Studies done on animals don't necessarily apply to humans. Likewise, those done on males may not apply to females. And so on.

➤ Consider how many and how people were studied. If only a small number of people were studied, the chances that the results don't apply to the general population are high. What was the dietary treatment in the study? Were people fed abnormally large amounts of food, more than anyone would eat? Unusual treatments give unusual results.

➤ Consider the original source of the information. Was the study published in a peer-reviewed scientific journal? Or is it based on personal testimony alone? Unlike scientists and health professionals, purveyors of quackery do not subject their products to the scrutiny of scientific research.

➤ Beware of promotions for a single product claimed to be effective for a wide variety of problems.

Above all, if a report suggests any action that goes beyond a well-balanced diet, such as taking large amounts of supplements, explore the pros and cons of the recommendation. One of the easiest ways to do that is to seek the advice of a health professional knowledgeable about diet and health, such as a registered dietitian.

Scientists have made great strides in understanding the substances in food and how they affect our health. Still, more research is needed to determine everything that is in our food that contributes to health. Vitamins, minerals, and dietary supplements can be a valuable part of a healthful diet for many people, but they cannot take the place of proper food choices. The best route to health is eating a varied, well-balanced diet.

Appendix One

What You Need to Know About Vitamins

OUR BODIES NEED at least 13 vitamins to function. The following pages include brief summaries about what each vitamin does; what happens if you don't get enough; what happens if you get too much; and what foods are good sources for that vitamin. (Appendix 2 contains similar information for minerals.)

Also included here are the most recent Recommended Dietary Allowances (RDAs) or Adequate Intakes (AIs) for each vitamin. These recommendations are scientifically determined to provide a "margin of safety" that, in essence, assures the amounts are high enough to meet the needs of almost everyone, while also ensuring they are not so high as to cause harm in some people. Supplements that exceed these amounts are not generally recommended. The RDAs and AIs are intended to be goals for average daily intakes over time, not necessarily for single days.

In addition, there are a few vitamins and minerals for which "Estimated Safe and Adequate Daily Dietary Intakes" (ESADDI) have been set. It's clear that these vitamins and minerals are essential to good health, but we don't know enough yet to establish RDAs for them. As our understanding of their function advances, these vitamins and minerals may someday achieve RDA status. For example, vitamin K and selenium were at one time listed in the ESADDI table, but now have established RDAs. Caution: The higher amounts listed in the ranges for vitamins and minerals in the ESADDI table should not be habitually exceeded because the toxic level may be only several times the usual intake. Play it safe by being moderate if you use supplements that contain these vitamins and minerals.

Fat-Soluble Vitamins

Vitamin A

Functions—Vitamin A helps you see normally in the dark and promotes the growth and health of all body cells and tissues. It also protects against infection by keeping the skin and tissues in the mouth, stomach, intestines, and respiratory, genital, and urinary tracts healthy.

Deficiency problems—If you don't get enough vitamin A, you can suffer night blindness, other eye problems, dry, scaly skin, problems with reproduction, and poor growth.

Food sources—You get vitamin A in two ways from food. In animal foods, it's found as retinol (preformed vitamin A). Sources include liver, fish oil, eggs, milk fortified with vitamin A, and other vitamin A-fortified foods. In plants, it comes from carotenoids, such as beta carotene, that your body converts to vitamin A, if needed. Carotenoids are found in red, yellow, orange, and many dark-green leafy vegetables or in fruits such as spinach, collards, kale, mustard greens, turnip greens, broccoli, carrots, peaches, pumpkin, red peppers, sweet potatoes, and cantaloupe.

If you get too much—Too much vitamin A can cause birth defects during pregnancy; the Food and Nutrition Board recommends avoiding supplemental preformed vitamin A (retinol) during the first trimester of pregnancy. Excess intakes may also cause headaches, vomiting, double vision, hair loss, bone abnormalities, and liver damage. Excess usually only comes from supplements, not food (although it can come from eating large amounts of liver). Excess carotenoids from foods do not cause problems, although they may color the skin orange. The usefulness and safety of beta-carotene supplements is questionable (see "Focus on...Antioxidants," page 20).

Recommended Dietary Allowances, Vitamin A

microgram
retinol equivalents (RE)

Infants (0–12 mos)	375
Children (1–3 yrs).	400
(4–6 yrs)	500
(7–10 yrs)	700
Males (11+ yrs).	1000
Females (11+ yrs)	800
Pregnant	800
Lactating (1st 6 mos)	1300
Lactating (2nd 6 mos).	1200

Vitamin D (calciferol)

Functions—Vitamin D promotes the absorption of calcium and phosphorus and helps deposit these minerals in bones and teeth to make them strong.

Deficiency problems—If you don't get enough, in older years you may have greater loss of bone mass (osteoporosis) and risk of osteomalacia (softening of the bones). Children can develop rickets, or defective bone growth. Fortified milk has virtually wiped out rickets in the United States.

Food sources—Vitamin D is known as the "sunshine vitamin" because your body can make it after sunlight, or ultraviolet light, hits the skin. Sunscreens interfere or block this process. Older people make vitamin D less efficiently in this way. Some people also face higher risks for deficiencies during winter, especially if they don't get outdoors much. Food sources include cheese, eggs, some fish (sardines and salmon), fortified milk, breakfast cereals, and margarine.

If you get too much—Too much vitamin D can lead to kidney stones or kidney damage, weak muscles and bones, excessive bleeding, and other problems. Excess amounts usually come from supplements, not food or exposure to sunlight. Supplements may not be advisable for children or adults who drink at least two glasses of vitamin D-fortified milk daily.

Adequate Intakes, Vitamin D

micrograms

Infants (0–6 mos) 5
(6–12 mos) 5
Children (1–10 yrs). 5
Males (11–24 yrs) 5
(25–50 yrs) 5
(51–70 yrs) 10
(>70 yrs) 15
Females (11–24 yrs) 5
(25–50 yrs) 5
(51–70 yrs) 10
(>70 yrs) 15
Pregnant and Lactating 5

Vitamin E (tocopherol)

Functions—Vitamin E works as an antioxidant and, as such, may have a possible role in protecting against illnesses such as heart disease and some types of cancer.

Deficiency problems—Deficiencies are rare because vitamin E is so abundant in the food supply. Exceptions: Premature, very-low birthweight infants and people who don't absorb fat normally, and thus may not absorb enough vitamin E, may suffer nervous system effects.

Food sources—The best sources of vitamin E are vegetable oils and margarine, salad dressing, and other foods made from vegetable oils. Nuts, seeds, and wheat germ are also good sources. Leafy green vegetables provide smaller amounts.

If you get too much—Vitamin E is relatively nontoxic. High doses may interfere with vitamin K action and enhance the effect of some anticoagulant drugs.

Recommended Dietary Allowances, Vitamin E

milligrams
alpha-tocopherol
equivalents

Infants (0–6 mos) 3
(6–12 mos) 4
Children (1–3 yrs). 6
(4–10 yrs) 7

	milligrams alpha-tocopherol equivalents
Males (11+ yrs)	10
Females (11+ yrs)	8
Pregnant	10
Lactating (1st 6 mos)	12
Lactating (2nd 6 mos)	11

Vitamin K

Functions—Vitamin K helps blood to clot and stop bleeding.

Deficiency problems—Deficiencies create problems with blood coagulation. Deficiencies are rare, although prolonged use of antiobiotics can destroy intestinal bacteria that produce vitamin K.

Food sources—Intestinal bacteria produces some of the vitamin K you need. The best food sources include green leafy vegetables such as kale, parsley, spinach, and broccoli. Smaller amounts are found in milk and other dairy foods, meat, eggs, cereal, fruits, and other vegetables.

If you get too much—No symptoms have been observed from excessive amounts of vitamin K.

Recommended Dietary Allowances, Vitamin K

	micrograms
Infants (0–6 mos)	5
(6–12 mos)	10
Children (1–3 yrs)	15
(4–6 yrs)	20
(7–10 yrs)	30
Males (11–14 yrs)	45
(15–18 yrs)	65
(19–24 yrs)	70
(25+ yrs)	80
Females (11–14 yrs)	45
(15–18 yrs)	55
(19–24 yrs)	60
(25+ yrs)	65
Pregnant	65
Lactating	65

Water-Soluble Vitamins

Vitamin C (ascorbic acid)

Functions—Vitamin C plays a variety of roles in the body. It helps the body absorb iron from plant sources of food, and helps produce collagen, a connective tissue that holds muscles, bones, and other tissues together. It helps form and repair red blood cells, bones, and other tissues, and helps keep capillary walls and blood vessels firm, and so protects against bruising. Vitamin C is also important for healthy gums, to heal cuts and wounds, and to help protect from infection by keeping the immune system healthy.

Deficiency problems—A deficiency of vitamin C leads to scurvy, a disease that causes loose teeth, excessive bleeding, swollen gums, and improper wound healing. Scurvy is rare in the United States.

Food sources—Most vitamin C comes from plant sources of foods. Citrus fruits and many other fruits and vegetables, including berries, melons, peppers, many dark-green leafy vegetables, potatoes, and tomatoes supply significant amounts.

If you get too much—The most common side effects from excess vitamin C supplementation are diarrhea and gastrointestinal discomfort. Supplement use can also interfere with tests for blood sugar level.

Recommended Dietary Allowances, Vitamin C

	milligrams
Infants (0–6 mos)	30
(6–12 mos)	35
Children (1–3 yrs)	40
(4–10 yrs)	45
Males (11–14 yrs)	50
(15+ yrs)	60
Females (11–14 yrs)	50
(15+ yrs)	60
Pregnant	70
Lactating (1st 6 mos)	95
Lactating (2nd 6 mos)	90

Thiamin (vitamin B_1)

Functions—Thiamin helps all body cells produce energy from carbohydrates.

Deficiency problems—Because of enriched grain products, thiamin deficiencies are rare. Chronic alcoholics, however, are frequently low in thiamin, and suffer fatigue, weak muscles, and nerve damage as a result.

Food sources—Whole-grain and enriched grain products, such as bread, rice, pasta, tortillas, and fortified breakfast cereals. Pork, liver, and other organ meats also provide significant amounts.

If you get too much—Excess amounts of thiamin are excreted in the urine. Contrary to popular claims, extra amounts have no energy-boosting effect.

Recommended Dietary Allowances, Thiamin

	milligrams
Infants (0–5 mos)	0.2
(6–11 mos)	0.3
Children (1–3 yrs)	0.5
(4–8 yrs)	0.6
(9–13 yrs)	0.9
Males (14–70+ yrs)	1.2
Females (14–18 yrs)	1.0
(19–70+)	1.1
Pregnant	1.4
Lactating	1.5

Riboflavin (vitamin B_2)

Functions—Riboflavin helps all body cells produce energy. In addition to many other roles, it also helps change tryptophan (an amino acid) into niacin (another B vitamin).

Deficiency problems—Deficiencies are unlikely except in severely malnourished people. Symptoms include eye disorders (such as cataracts), dry and flaky skin, and a sore red tongue. Deficiencies do not cause hair loss.

Food sources—Milk and other dairy foods are major sources of riboflavin. Enriched bread, cereal, and other grain products, eggs, meat, green leafy vegetables, and nuts also supply riboflavin. Liver, kidney, and heart are excellent sources. Ultraviolet light, such as sunlight, destroys riboflavin. That's why milk is packed in opaque plastic or cardboard containers, not clear glass.

If you get too much—No problems have been linked to consuming too much riboflavin.

Recommended Dietary Allowances, Riboflavin

milligrams

Infants (0–5 mos)	0.3
(6–11 mos)	0.4
Children (1–3 yrs).	0.5
(4–8 yrs)	0.6
(9–13 yrs)	0.9
Males (14–70+ yrs)	1.3
Females (14–18 yrs)	1.0
(19–70+ yrs)	1.1
Pregnant	1.4
Lactating	1.6

Niacin

Functions—Niacin helps the body use sugars and fatty acids, and helps all body cells produce energy. It also helps enzymes function in the body.

Deficiency problems—Deficiencies are unlikely if you consume enough protein-rich foods. Symptoms include diarrhea, mental disorientation, and skin problems.

Food sources—Some niacin is produced in the body from tryptophan (an amino acid). Foods high in protein are also usually good sources of niacin: poultry, fish, beef, peanut butter, and legumes. Enriched and fortified grain products are also typically good sources.

If you get too much—Consuming excess amounts of nicotinic acid (one form of niacin), which usually only occurs with supplements, may cause flushed skin, liver damage, stomach ulcers, and high blood sugar.

Recommended Dietary Allowances, Niacin

milligrams

Infants (0–5 mos)	2
(6–11 mos)	3
Children (1–3 yrs)	6
(4–8 yrs)	8
(9–13 yrs)	12
Males (14–70+ yrs)	16
Females (14–70+ yrs)	14
Pregnant	18
Lactating	17

Vitamin B6 (pyridoxine)

Functions—Vitamin B6 helps the body make proteins, which are then used to make body cells. It also helps convert tryptophan (an amino acid) into niacin and serotonin (a brain chemical). Vitamin B6 also helps produce other body chemicals such as insulin, hemoglobin, and antibodies to fight infection.

Deficiency problems—Deficiencies can cause mental convulsions in infants, depression, nausea, and greasy, flaky skin.

Food sources—Chicken, fish, pork, liver, and kidney are the best sources. Whole grains, nuts, and legumes also supply pyridoxine.

If you get too much—Large doses of vitamin B6, taken for an extended period, can cause nerve damage.

Recommended Dietary Allowances, Vitamin B6

milligrams

Infants (0–5 mos)	0.1
(6–11 mos)	0.3
Children (1–3 yrs)	0.5
(4–8 yrs)	0.6
(9–13 yrs)	1.0
Males (14–50 yrs)	1.3
(51–70+ yrs)	1.7
Females (14–18 yrs)	1.2
(19–50 yrs)	1.3
(51–70+ yrs)	1.5
Pregnant	1.9
Lactating	2.0

Folate (folic acid)

Functions—Folate plays an essential role in producing DNA and RNA to make new body cells. It also works with vitamin B_{12} to form hemoglobin in red blood cells. Folic acid is the manmade form of folate.

Deficiency problems—Deficiencies impair normal cell division and growth. One type of anemia can result from a folate deficiency. Inadequate amounts of folic acid during the first trimester of pregnancy may increase the risk of delivering a baby with neural tube defects, including spina bifida (see "The Child-Bearing Years," page 36).

Food sources—Leafy vegetables, orange juice and some fruits, legumes, liver, yeast breads, and wheat germ. Bread, cereal, rice, and pasta products are fortified with folic acid.

If you get too much—Too much folate can interfere with medications and cause convulsions in people with epilepsy. It can also mask vitamin B_{12} deficiencies, leading to permanent nerve damage if not treated with vitamin B_{12}.

Recommended Dietary Allowances, Folate

micrograms

Infants (0–5 mos)	65
(6–12 mos)	80
Children (1–3 yrs)	150
(4–8 yrs)	200
(9–13 yrs)	300
Males (14–70+ yrs)	400
Females (14–70+ yrs)	400
Pregnant	600
Lactating	500

Vitamin B_{12} (cobalamin)

Functions—Vitamin B_{12} works with folate to make red blood cells. It also serves in every body cell as a vital part of many body chemicals, and helps the body use fatty acids and some amino acids.

Deficiency problems—Deficiencies can result in anemia, fatigue, nerve damage, a smooth tongue, or very sensitive skin. B_{12} deficiencies can be hidden when extra folate is taken to treat or prevent anemia. Strict vegetarians who eat no animal products and their infants are the most likely to develop vitamin B_{12} deficiencies. People who do not absorb vitamin B_{12} may also be deficient. Older adults (over 50 years) should get most of their vitamin B_{12} from foods fortified with this vitamin, such as breakfast cereals, or from a B_{12}-containing supplement.

Food sources—Vitamin B_{12} is found in animal products, including meat, fish, poultry, eggs, milk, and other dairy foods, and some fortified foods.

If you get too much—No symptoms are known from excessive intake of vitamin B_{12}. But research does not show taking extra vitamin B_{12} boosts energy, either.

Recommended Dietary Allowances, Vitamin B_{12}

	micrograms
Infants (0–5 mos)	0.4
(6–11 mos)	0.5
Children (1–3 yrs)	0.9
(4–8 yrs)	1.2
(9–13 yrs)	1.8
Males (14–70+ yrs)	2.4
Females (14–70+ yrs)	2.4
Pregnant	2.6
Lactating	2.8

Biotin

Functions—Biotin helps all body cells produce energy. It also helps metabolize protein, fat, and carbohydrate in food.

Deficiency problems—Deficiencies are rare in healthy people who eat a balanced diet. Symptoms include heart abnormalities, appetite loss, fatigue, depression, and dry skin.

Food sources—Biotin is found in a wide variety of foods. Eggs, liver, yeast breads, and cereals are among the best sources.

If you get too much—No negative effects have been reported due to consuming too much biotin.

Adequate Intakes, Biotin

	micrograms
Infants (0–5 mos)	5
(6–11 mos)	6
Children (1–3 yrs)	8
(4–8 yrs)	12
(9–13 yrs)	20
Males (14–18 yrs)	25
(19–70+ yrs)	30
Females (14–18 yrs)	25
(19–70+ yrs)	30
Pregnant	30
Lactating	35

Pantothenic Acid

Functions—Pantothenic acid helps all body cells produce energy. It also helps metabolize protein, fat, and carbohydrate in food.

Deficiency problems—Deficiencies are rare in healthy people who eat a balanced diet.

Food sources—Pantothenic acid is widely available in food. Meat, poultry, fish, whole-grain cereals, and legumes are among the best sources. Milk, vegetables, and fruits also contain varying amounts.

If you get too much—Too much pantothenic acid may cause occasional diarrhea and water retention.

Adequate Intakes, Pantothenic Acid

	milligrams
Infants (0–5 mos)	1.7
(6–11 mos)	1.8
Children (1–3 yrs)	2
(4–8 yrs)	3
(9–13 yrs)	4
Males (14–70+ yrs)	5
Females (14–70+ yrs)	5
Pregnant	6
Lactating	7

Choline

Functions—Classified as a natural food component, recommendations for choline intake were released for the first time in 1998. Choline appears to play a role in many body processes, including maintaining liver function. However, it's questionable whether a dietary supply of choline is really needed at all stages of life. Our bodies may be able to produce enough during some stages.

Deficiency problems—none known

Food sources—Choline is widely distributed in food. Milk, liver, eggs, and peanuts are especially good sources.

Adequate Intakes, Choline

	milligrams
Infants (0–5 mos)	125
(6–11 mos)	150
Children (1–3 yrs)	200
(4–8 yrs)	250
(9–13 yrs)	375
Males (14–70+ yrs)	550
Females (14–18 yrs)	400
(19–70+ yrs)	425
Pregnant	450
Lactating	550

What You Need to Know About Minerals

AS MENTIONED EARLIER, we need at least 13 vitamins to function. Fifteen minerals have also been identified as needed by our bodies. The following pages includes brief summaries about what each mineral does, what happens if you don't get enough; what happens if you get too much, and what foods are good sources for that mineral. (Appendix 1 contains similar information for vitamins.)

Also included here are the most recent Recommended Dietary Allowances (RDAs) or Adequate Intakes (AIs) for each mineral. Again, these amounts are scientifically determined to provide a "margin of safety" that, in essence, assures the amounts are high enough to meet the needs of almost everyone, while also ensuring they are not so high as to cause harm in some people. Supplements that exceed these amounts are not generally recommended. The RDAs and AIs are intended to be goals for average daily intakes over time, not necessarily for single days.

In addition to RDAs, there are a few vitamins and minerals for which "Estimated Safe and Adequate Daily Dietary Intakes" (ESADDI) have been set. These vitamins and minerals are essential to good health, but we don't know enough yet about them to establish their RDAs. With more research, though, these vitamins and minerals may someday achieve RDA status. Caution: The higher amounts listed in the ranges for vitamins and minerals in the ESADDI table should not be habitually exceeded because the toxic level may be only several times the usual intake. Play it safe by being moderate if you use supplements that contain these vitamins and minerals.

Major Minerals
Calcium

Functions—Calcium builds bones, both in length and strength, and helps keep them strong by slowing the rate of bone loss as you age. Calcium also helps muscles contract, including the heart, plays a role in normal nerve function, and helps blood clot when bleeding.

Deficiency problems—Insufficient calcium affects bone density, increasing the risk for osteoporosis.

Food sources—Good sources of calcium include milk and milk products such as cheese, yogurt, frozen yogurt; some dark-green leafy vegetables (kale, broccoli, bok choy); fish with edible bones; and tofu made with calcium sulfate. Many foods are fortified with calcium, such as some brands of orange juice, bread, and soy milk.

If you get too much—Too much calcium over a prolonged period can cause constipation, kidney stones, and poor kidney function. Excess calcium may also interfere with the absorption of other minerals such as iron and zinc. Excess amounts are only consumed via supplements, not from drinking milk. More than 2500 milligrams daily is not recommended.

Adequate Intakes, Calcium

milligrams

Infants (0–6 mos) 210
(6–12 mos) 270
Children (1–3 yrs) 500
(4–8 yrs) 800
Males (9–18 yrs) 1300
(19–50 yrs) 1000
(51–70+ yrs) 1200
Females (9–18 yrs) 1300
(19–50 yrs) 1000
(51–70+ yrs) 1200
Pregnant and lactating (<18 yrs) . 1300
(19–50 yrs) 1000

Phosphorus

Functions—Phosphorus helps every body cell produce energy and acts as a main regulator of energy metabolism in body organs. It's a major component of bones and teeth (second only to calcium), and makes up part of DNA and RNA, which are the body's master plan for cell growth and repair.

Deficiency problems—Deficiencies are rare except for small premature babies who consume only breast milk, or for people taking an aluminum hydroxide-containing antacid for long periods. Symptoms include bone loss, weakness, loss of appetite, and pain.

Food sources—Almost all foods contain phosphorus. Protein-rich foods (milk, meat, poultry, fish, and eggs) are best sources. Legumes and nuts rank next. Even bread and baked goods contain phosphorus.

If you get too much—Too much phosphorus may lower calcium levels in the blood and increase bone loss if calcium intake is low. Excess dietary phosphorus does not appear to be a problem in U.S. diets.

Recommended Dietary Allowances, Phosphorus

	milligrams
Infants (0–6 mos)	100
(6–12 mos)	275
Children (1–3 yrs)	460
(4–8 yrs)	500
(9–13 yrs)	1250
Males (14–18 yrs)	1250
(19–70+ yrs)	700
Females (14–18 yrs)	1250
(19–70+ yrs)	700
Pregnant and lactating (<18 yrs)	1250
(19–50 yrs)	700

Magnesium

Functions—Magnesium is an important part of more than 300 enzymes, which regulate many body functions, including energy production and muscle contractions. It also helps maintain nerve and muscle cells, and is a component of bones.

What You Need to Know About Minerals

Deficiency problems—Deficiencies occur in diseases where the body cannot absorb magnesium properly. Symptoms include irregular heartbeat, nausea, weakness, and mental derangement.

Food sources—Magnesium is found in all kinds of foods in varying amounts. Best sources include legumes, nuts, and whole grains. Green vegetables are good sources.

If you get too much—Too much magnesium can cause nausea, vomiting, low blood pressure, and heart problems. Excess amounts from food are unlikely to cause harm unless kidney disease prevents magnesium from being excreted.

Recommended Dietary Allowances, Magnesium

	milligrams
Infants (0–6 mos)	30
(6–12 mos)	75
Children (1–3 yrs)	80
(4–8 yrs)	130
(9–13 yrs)	240
Males (14–18 yrs)	410
(19–30 yrs)	400
(31–70+ yrs)	420
Females (14–18 yrs)	360
(19–30 yrs)	310
(31–70+ yrs)	320
Pregnant (<18 yrs)	400
(19–30 yrs)	350
(31–50)	360
Lactating (<18 yrs)	360
(19–30 yrs)	310
(31–50)	320

Trace Minerals

Chromium

Functions—Chromium works with insulin to help the body use glucose (blood sugar).

Deficiency problems—Deficiency symptoms can resemble diabetes, including impaired glucose tolerance and nerve damage.

Food sources—Good sources include meat, whole grains, and nuts.

If you get too much—The toxicity of chromium appears to

be low. But potential side effects from high doses from supplements have some experts calling for more research. Excess chromium from supplements is stored in the body.

Estimated Safe and Adequate Daily Dietary Intakes, Chromium

	micrograms
Infants (0–6 mos)	10–40
(6–12 mos)	20–60
Children (1–3 yrs)	20–80
(4–6 yrs)	30–120
(7+ yrs)	50–200
Adults	50–200

Copper

Functions—Copper helps make hemoglobin, to carry oxygen in blood. It's also a part of many body enzymes, and helps all body cells produce energy.

Deficiency problems—Deficiencies rarely result from lack of copper in diet, but instead from genetic problems or consuming too much zinc. Excess zinc from dietary supplements can hinder copper absorption.

Food sources—Organ meats, especially liver, seafood, nuts, and seeds are good sources of copper. Cooking in copper pots also increases copper content of foods.

If you get too much—Too much copper can cause nausea, vomiting, diarrhea, coma, and liver damage. Harmful effects of copper from dietary sources are extremely rare in the United States.

Estimated Safe and Adequate Daily Dietary Intakes, Copper

	milligrams
Infants (0–6 mos)	0.4–0.6
(6–12 mos)	0.6–0.7
Children (1–3 yrs)	0.7–1
(4–6 yrs)	1–1.5
(7–10 yrs)	1–2
(11+ yrs)	1.5–2.5
Adults	1.5–3

Fluoride

Functions—Fluoride helps harden tooth enamel, protecting teeth from decay. It may also protect against osteoporosis by strengthening bones.

Deficiency problems—Deficiencies may result in weak tooth enamel.

Food sources—The only significant food sources of fluoride are tea (especially if made with fluoridated water) and fish with edible bones, such as canned salmon. Many communities add fluoride to the water supply. Use fluoride supplements under a doctor's direction. Some types of cooking utensils, such as Teflon with its fluoride-containing polymer, can increase the fluoride content of food.

If you get too much—Too much fluoride can mottle, or stain, otherwise healthy teeth. Excess fluoride can also lead to brittle bones and increase the frequency of bone fractures.

Adequate Intake, Fluoride

	milligrams
Infants (0–6 mos)	0.01
(6–12 mos)	0.5
Children (1–3 yrs)	0.7
(4–8 yrs)	1
(9–13 yrs)	2
Males (14–18 yrs)	3
(19–70+ yrs)	4
Females (14–70+ yrs)	3
Pregnant and lactating	3

Iodine

Functions—Iodine is part of thyroxin (thyroid hormone), which regulates the rate at which the body uses energy.

Deficiency problems—Deficiency interferes with thyroxin production, slowing the rate at which the body burns energy. Symptoms include weight gain and goiter (enlarged thyroid gland). Use of iodized salt has virtually eliminated iodine deficiency as a cause of goiter in the United States.

Food sources—Iodine is found naturally in saltwater fish and foods grown near coastal areas. Small amounts of iodine are also found in foods as a result of the use of iodine-containing disinfectants and dough conditioners. To assure adequate iodine in the diet, however, iodine is added to salt. One-half teaspoon of salt provides approximately the RDA.

If you get too much—Goiter can also occur when people consume too much iodine—but not at levels consumed in the United States.

Recommended Dietary Allowances per day, Iodine
micrograms

Infants (0–6 mos) 40
(6–12 mos) 50
Children (1–3 yrs). 70
(4–6 yrs) 90
(7–10 yrs) 120
Males (11+ yrs) 150
Females (11+ yrs) 150
Pregnant 175
Lactating. 200

Iron

Functions—Iron is an essential part of hemoglobin, which carries oxygen to body cells.

Deficiency problems—Iron deficiency can lead to anemia, fatigue, and infections. Deficiencies are more common among women with regular menstrual periods.

Food sources—Iron is found in foods of both animal and plant sources. Some iron from animal sources ("heme" iron) is better absorbed than plant ("non-heme") sources. (See "Focus on… Iron," page 24.)

If you get too much—Adult iron supplements can be harmful for children; seek immediate medical attention if they accidentally take such supplements. Iron supplements should also not be taken by men, postmenopausal women, and people with a genetic problem called hemochromatosis.

Recommended Dietary Allowances, Iron

	milligrams
Infants (0–6 mos)	6
(6–12 mos)	10
Children (1–10 yrs)	10
Males (11–18 yrs)	12
(19+ yrs)	10
Females (11–50 yrs)	15
(51+ yrs)	10
Pregnant	30
Lactating	15

Manganese

Functions—Manganese is part of many body enzymes.

Deficiency problems—Deficiencies are rare because manganese is widely distributed in foods.

Food sources—Whole grain products are the best sources of manganese, along with some fruits and vegetables such as pineapple, kale, and strawberries. Tea is also a good source.

If you get too much—Consuming harmful levels of manganese from food is very rare. Nervous system damage has been seen in workers exposed to manganese dust or fumes.

Estimated Safe and Adequate Daily Dietary Intakes, Manganese

	milligrams
Infants (0–6 mos)	0.3–0.6
(6–12 mos)	0.6–1
Children (1–3 yrs)	1–1.5
(4–6 yrs)	1.5–2
(7–10 yrs)	2–3
(11+ yrs)	2–5
Adults	2–5

Molybdenum

Functions—Molybdenum works with riboflavin to incorporate iron into hemoglobin for red blood cells. It is also part of many body enzymes.

Deficiency problems—Deficiencies are rare with a normal diet.

Food sources—Molybdenum is found in milk, legumes, breads, and grain products.

If you get too much—Too much molybdenum may interfere with your body's ability to use copper.

Estimated Safe and Adequate Daily Dietary Intakes, Molybdenum

	micrograms
Infants (0–6 mos)	15–30
(6–12 mos)	20–40
Children (1–3 yrs)	25–50
(4–6 yrs)	30–75
(7–10 yrs)	50–150
(11+ yrs)	75–250
Adults	75–250

Selenium

Functions—Selenium works as an antioxidant with vitamin E, to protect body cells from damage that may lead to cancer, heart disease, and other health problems. It also aids cell growth.

Deficiency problems—Deficiencies may affect the heart.

Food sources—Seafood, liver, kidney, and other meats are the richest sources of selenium. Grain products and seeds also contain selenium, but the amount depends on the content of the soil in which they are grown.

If you get too much—Too much selenium can cause nausea, vomiting, abdominal pain, diarrhea, nail and hair changes, nerve damage, fatigue, and irritability.

Recommended Dietary Allowances, Selenium

	micrograms
Infants (0–6 mos)	10
(6–12 mos)	15
Children (1–6 yrs)	20
(7–10 yrs)	30
Males (11–14 yrs)	40
(15–18 yrs)	50
(19+ yrs)	70
Females (11–14 yrs)	45
(15–18 yrs)	50
(19+ yrs)	55
Pregnant	65
Lactating	75

Zinc

Functions—Zinc is essential for growth. It promotes cell reproduction, tissue growth and repair, and wound healing. It forms part of more than 70 body enzymes, and helps the body use carbohydrate, protein, and fat.

Deficiency problems—Deficiency can cause birth defects and retarded growth during childhood. Symptoms also include appetite loss, decreased sense of taste and smell, skin changes, and reduced resistance to infection.

Food sources—Meat, liver, and seafood are the best sources of zinc. Whole-grain products, wheat bran, legumes, and soybeans are good sources.

If you get too much—Excess zinc intake only occurs with supplements. It can cause gastrointestinal irritation, vomiting, reduced HDL ("good" cholesterol) levels, and can interfere with copper absorption and immune function.

Recommended Dietary Allowances, Zinc

	milligrams
Infants (0–12 mos)	5
Children (1–10 yrs)	10
Males (11+ yrs)	15
Females (11+ yrs)	12
Pregnant	15
Lactating (1st 6 mos)	19
Lactating (2nd 6 mos)	16

Major Minerals: Electrolytes
Chloride

Functions—Chloride helps regulate fluids in and out of body cells. It forms part of stomach acid to help digest food and absorb nutrients. It also helps transmit nerve impulses.

Deficiency problems—Deficiencies are rare because chloride is found in table salt. Heavy, persistent sweating, chronic diarrhea or vomiting, trauma, or kidney disease may cause deficiencies.

Food sources—The best source is table salt (1/4 teaspoon contains 750 mg of chloride). Minimum requirements are easily met with everyday food choices.

If you get too much—Excess chloride may be linked to high blood pressure in chloride-sensitive people. More study is needed to clearly establish the relationship between chloride and blood pressure.

Potassium

Functions—Potassium helps regulate fluids and mineral balance in and out of body cells. It also helps maintain normal blood pressure, transmit nerve impulses, and contract muscles.

Deficiency problems—Prolonged vomiting, diarrhea, laxative use, or kidney problems can result in deficiencies of potassium. Symptoms include weakness, appetite loss, nausea, and fatigue. Supplements may be necessary for people taking high blood pressure medication. Check with your doctor.

Food sources—Potassium is found in a wide range of foods, especially fruits, vegetables, fresh meat, poultry, and fish. Particularly good sources include apricots, avocados, bananas, cantaloupe, grapefruit, honeydew, kiwi, oranges, prunes, strawberries, potatoes, tomatoes, and dried fruits. Most people easily meet minimum requirements with varied food choices.

If you get too much—Excess amounts of potassium are usually excreted. If they can't be (as in people with some types of kidney disease), heart problems can occur.

Sodium

Functions—Sodium helps regulate movement of fluids in and out of body cells. It also helps transmit nerve impulses, regulate blood pressure, and relax muscles.

Deficiency problems—Deficiencies are unlikely except with chronic diarrhea or vomiting, or kidney problems. Symptoms include nausea, dizziness, and muscle cramps.

Food sources—Processed foods account for about 75 percent of the sodium we eat. Another 25 percent comes from table salt (1/4 teaspoon contains 500 mg of sodium). A small amount occurs naturally in food. Minimum requirements are easily met by everyday food choices.

If you get too much—Healthy people excrete excess sodium. But some kidney diseases interfere with sodium excretion, leading to fluid retention and swelling. Sodium sensitive people may experience high blood pressure eating a daily diet that contains high levels of sodium.

Index